Managing the Clinical
Drug Development Process

DRUGS AND THE PHARMACEUTICAL SCIENCES

A Series of Textbooks and Monographs

edited by
James Swarbrick
School of Pharmacy
University of North Carolina
Chapel Hill, North Carolina

Managing the Clinical Drug Development Process

David M. Cocchetto
Glaxo Inc.
Research Triangle Park, North Carolina

Ronald V. Nardi
Parke-Davis Pharmaceutical Research Division
Warner-Lambert Company
Ann Arbor, Michigan

Marcel Dekker, Inc.   **New York • Basel • Hong Kong**

FIRST INDIAN REPRINT, 2014

Library of Congress Cataloging-in-Publication Data

Cocchetto, David M.
    Managing the clinical drug development process / David M.
Cocchetto, Ronald V. Nardi.
        p.   cm. -- (Drugs and the pharmaceutical sciences; v. 51)
    Includes bibliographical references and index.
    ISBN 0-8247-8595-9 (alk. paper)
        1. Drugs--Testing. 2. Drugs--Research--Management. 3. Drugs--
-Effectiveness--Evaluation. I. Nardi, Ronald V. II. Title.
III. Series.
        [DNLM: 1. Clinical Trials. 2. Drug Industry--organization &
administration. W1 DR8938.51 / QV 771 C659m]
    RM301.27.C631992
    615'.19--dc20
    DNLM/DLC
    for Library of Congress   91-30971
                                                                        CIP

MARCEL DEKKER, INC.
270 Madison Avenue, New York, New York 10016

Printed and bound in India by Bhavish Graphics.

FOR SALE IN SOUTH ASIA ONLY

We dedicate this book to examples of personal sacrifice and professional inspiration. Personal sacrifice and great tolerance have been shown by our wives, Linda and Michele. Professional inspiration is found in the many patients who volunteer to participate in clinical studies of drugs with unknown benefits and uncharacterized risks. Their faith, hope, and trust in their doctors, clinical scientists, and protections afforded by the regulatory process must be respected and guarded as an invaluable natural resource.

Preface

A successful clinical drug development process must integrate three distinct types of expertise. First, pharmacotherapeutic expertise is needed to develop a drug in an area of medical therapeutics where a true therapeutic need and market do, in fact, exist. Second, drug development expertise is needed to perform the planning, initiation, conduct, completion, analysis, and reporting of results from the clinical trials executed to develop the substantial evidence of safety and efficacy of the drug in man. Third, management expertise is needed to plan, organize, staff, lead, and control the administrative aspects of this complex managerial activity. Functional integration of these three types of expertise is essential to achieving efficient and successful clinical drug development.

We decided to prepare this book for three reasons. First, our goal was to write an integrated series of chapters on application of drug development expertise and management expertise to clinical drug development. We attempted to present an integrated view of lessons learned from several historical drug development programs. Our second goal was to describe the key aspects of drug development expertise. Many scientists, clinicians, R&D administrators, and project managers do not fully appreciate that expertise in clinical drug development is distinct from expertise in pharmacotherapeutics or medicine. In order to illuminate the unique nature of drug development expertise, we focused several chapters on application of the principles of dose-response and characterization of the benefit/risk ratio of a new drug. An understanding of the methods of benefit/risk assessment can be translated into action plans for managers of clinical research.

This leads to the third goal for this book, namely, to discuss management of clinical research. Management is classically defined as the process of planning, organizing, staffing, leading, and controlling. Managers must perform these functions despite being surrounded by rapid changes in the pharmaceutical industry. These changes are the result of industrial consolidation, internationalization of the clinical research process, and dramatic economic pressures for more rapid new product development, to name a few major trends. Any one of these changes could distract attention from thoughtful, scientific evaluation of a new chemical entity progressing through the development process. We discuss the management challenge of maintaining continuity in drug development programs. A comparative summary is presented of the basic project management systems that have been applied to clinical drug development. The different management implications of the different portions of the pharmaceutical business that are intellect-limited, as opposed to resource-limited, are discussed. Finally, we consider some of the management challenges faced by clinical researchers who must interact effectively with marketing personnel.

Our intent throughout this book was to capture a variety of fundamental ideas about clinical development of drugs. We hope to stimulate the reader to think about issues in benefit/risk assessment, the sliding scale of benefits and risks for different diseases, the role of the recent expansion in treatment use of investigational drugs, critical mass, project team concepts, and research equity as a basis for drug development. The final unit of this book presents a view of the past, present, and future of clinical research. The past includes the very young history and rapid evolution of the laws and regulations governing clinical drug development in the United States. The segments on the present and future discuss our observations regarding current trends and controversies, as well as future directions of clinical drug development.

Several items presented in this book are unique. As drug developers, we have found this information useful in our own activities and to our colleagues. We hope readers find it useful too. For example, the tables in Chapter 1 summarize the numbers of drugs approved, by therapeutic importance by FDA categories, over the decade of the 1980s. Certainly, this information is publicly available, but it has not previously been summarized in this form. Chapter 4 presents an overview of the principles of dose-response applied specifically to clinical drug development. Chapter 5 expresses in words in sliding-scale concept of benefit/risk, e.g., the intuitive notion that higher drug-associated toxicity can be acceptable if the drug is a treatment for diseases with higher morbidity or mortality. This concept is regularly seen in use but has not been discussed in the drug development literature. Chapter 6 presents an integrated discussion of the different ways for treatment use of an investigational drug. In view of the many recent new and proposed regulations affecting treatment use, this book is the first to present a comparison of the features of these different approaches with a summary of the regulatory conditions for each approach. In Chapter 9, intellect-limited projects (e.g., certain R&D activities) and resource-limited projects (e.g., manufacturing) are contrasted in order to remind drug developers that intellectual limitation is the rate-limiting component of each R&D project. Chapter 10 draws information from some literature on organizational communication to describe the common communication difficulties between clinical research and marketing groups. Chapter 11 reviews the lessons of the past from the viewpoint of the various public health crises that preceded each piece of new federal legislation. We believe this book provides a comprehensive summary, in a manner understandable to R&D personnel, of the laws affecting clinical drug development.

This book is not without controversy. Most of the controversy will arise in discussion of our views of the lessons learned from the past. We learned these lessons based on our interpretation of previous clinical drug development programs. We do not provide a collection of tried and true methods of drug development because, we argue, no such "universal methods" survive even short periods of time in the dynamic environments of research and medicine.

We hope the readers of this book find it thought-provoking and unique. The primary audience for this book is scientists and physicians who work at a project-leader level in clinical drug development. We also hope that some of these ideas contribute to successful clinical development of safe and effective new drugs to benefit the many patients with inadequately treated or untreated diseases.

David M. Cocchetto
Ronald V. Nardi

Contents

Part Three
ISSUES IN MANAGING CLINICAL DRUG DEVELOPMENT

Managing the Clinical Drug Development Process

part one

Introduction to Clinical Drug Development

1
Basic Concepts of Clinical Drug Development

> The only sure foundations of medicine are, an intimate knowledge of the human body, and observation on the effects of medicinal substances on that.
>
> *Thomas Jefferson*

I. INTRODUCTION

Clinical drug development is the process by which new chemicals progress from preclinical evaluations to regulatory approval for safe and effective use in man for the cure, mitigation, or prevention of disease. This process operates with multiple inputs from different technical fields, including chemical synthesis, pharmacologic evaluation, toxicologic evaluation, pharmaceutical formulation, analytical chemistry, clinical pharmacology, medicine, statistics, and epidemiology. These inputs are used to produce a clinical drug development plan. This plan is a dynamic document which evolves as increasing knowledge of the drug is obtained. Successful growth and execution of the plan should result in 1 of 2 successful outcomes: (1) approved drug or (2) justifiable termination of development after the least investment possible.

Some of the principal ideas that we will expand on in this book are that (1) the diverse inputs to the clinical drug development process necessitate formation of a multidisciplinary critical mass project team to drive the development process, (2) many of the most effective actions of project teams are to recommend termination of a drug's development as soon as sufficient negative evidence is available, and (3) truly exciting therapeutic advances usually follow a major breakthrough in our understanding of the pathophysiology of target diseases.

The Pharmaceutical Manufacturers Association has estimated that development of a new chemical entity costs approximately $125,000,000 [1]. To place some perspective on that cost, it can be viewed by the "rule of 50" as the total salary earned by 50 people working 50 years for $50,000 per person per year! This extraordinarily high cost has made drug discovery a business for fully committed enterprises. High cost is surely one factor fueling the consolidation of companies in this industry.

II. WHY DRUGS FAIL TO ATTAIN APPROVAL

Miller and colleagues [2] have provided an elegant distillation of years of experience to provide a list of the four predominant areas of deficiencies responsible for failure of a drug to attain approval from FDA. The interested reader is urged to consult that paper since only a summary is provided here. Drugs fail to attain approval for the following four reasons: (1) inadequate characterization of dose-response profiles, both in terms of peak response and time course of response during a dosage interval; (2) flaws in study design or the drug development plan providing inappropriate studies, studies that are difficult to interpret, or studies based on unfounded assumptions; (3) inadequate characterization of the benefit/risk profile; and (4) inadequate proof that the quality of life of the target patient group is improved with therapy. Describing approaches to preventing each of these potential deficiencies is one goal of this book.

III. PREREQUISITES TO SUCCESSFUL CLINICAL DRUG DEVELOPMENT

We have tried to distill a list of the essential intellectual prerequisites to successful clinical development of a drug. Table 1 summarizes eight essential factors. These eight factors can be divided into two subgroups, i.e., one subgroup of four factors dependent on the target disease and a second subgroup of four factors dependent on the specific drug. By disease-dependent, we mean some increased knowledge of some aspect of the pathophysiology of the target disease. For successful development of new drugs for a disease, clinical scientists must understand the natural history of the target disease, the differences among various subpopulations of patients with the target disease, characteristics of patients that may be predictive of good response versus poor response to therapeutic intervention, and quantifiable indices of the disease that can be used as measures of respon-

Table 1. Items needed for successful clinical development of a drug.

Items Dependent on the Target Disease:

1. a defined target disease with known natural history
2. a defined patient population with the target disease
3. a set of patient characteristics that render the patients potentially responsive to therapeutic interventions
4. defined and quantifiable measures of the disease which are known to change over a sufficiently rapid timeframe to enable use in prospective studies and known to be sensitive in a dose-related manner to therapeutic interventions

Items Dependent on the Drug:

5. a profile of non-limiting preclinical toxicological findings
6. a pharmaceutical formulation which provides a means to adequately deliver the drug to the site of action
7. methods to characterize the pharmacodynamic and pharmacokinetic properties of the drug in man
8. defined and quantifiable measures of the non-disease-related effects of the drug

siveness. Each of these factors is *independent* of the specific drug under study, but dependent on knowledge of the target disease.

Some examples may clarify the types of disease-dependent knowledge referred to in items 1-4 of Table 1. A new therapeutic approach to treatment of hypercholesterolemia was envisioned after scientists obtained the disease-specific knowledge that the enzyme HMGCoA reductase governs the rate-limiting step in cholesterol biosynthesis. This knowledge was a critical precursor to the design and chemical synthesis of selective enzyme inhibitors such as lovastatin. In the 1970s, microbiologists began to understand the role of DNA gyrase in the life processes of various bacteria, as well as defining the A subunit of DNA gyrase as a primary target of some early quinolones. This greater understanding ultimately facilitated development of several expanded-spectrum quinolone antibiotics for use in man. Endoscopic methods provided direct visualization and evaluation of gastrointestinal lesions, including duodenal and gastric ulcers. Availability of endoscopy enabled a detailed, semi-quantitative characterization of the esophageal lesions in some patients with GERD (gastroesophageal reflux disease). This ability to endoscopically characterize disease-related lesions was an essential precursor to development of the H-2-antagonists for ulcer disease and ranitidine for treatment of GERD. These and other examples are summarized in Table 2. Clearly, aggressive and careful discovery and

Table 2. Examples of advances in disease-dependent knowledge that preceded development of clinically useful new drugs.

Disease	Advance	Old Therapies	New Therapy (year approved by FDA)
Hypercholesterolemia	knowledge of properties of HMGCoA reductase	adsorbents (e.g., cholestyramine) clofibrate gemfibrozil	lovastatin (1987)
Selected bacterial infections	knowledge of roles of DNA gyrase	beta-lactam antibiotics aminoglycosides macrolides tetracyclines	quinolone antibiotics: ciprofloxacin (1987) norfloxacin (1986)
Duodenal ulcer (DU), gastric ulcer (GU), and GERD	endoscopic characterization of gastrointestinal lesions	antacids	cimetidine (DU & GU; 1977) ranitidine (DU & GU; 1983) ranitidine (GERD; 1986)

Depression	role of serotonergic function in psychiatric diseases	tricyclic antidepressants MAO inhibitors	fluoxetine (1987)
Chemotherapy-induced emesis	role of serotonergic function in emesis	prochlorperazine metoclopramide tetrahydrocannabinol	selective 5HT antagonists: ondansetron (1991)
Diabetic retinopathy	knowledge of properties of aldose reductase	none	investigational drugs under development (e.g., ponalrestat)
AIDS	causative role of HTLV-III (HIV)	none	zidovudine (1987)
Leprosy	characterization of dapsone-resistant strains of *Mycobacterium leprae*	dapsone sulfoxone	clofazimine (1986)

characterization of key disease-related factors (e.g., a rate-limiting enzyme-catalyzed step or a neurochemical pathway previously not thought to be important in a certain disease process) can provide opportunities to subject these newly identified targets to therapeutic intervention with a novel new drug.

Successful clinical development of a drug also requires certain prerequisite knowledge that is dependent on the drug. Four drug-dependent factors were listed in Table 1. In order to progress in man, the drug must not possess any limiting findings in preclinical toxicology studies. The drug must possess physicochemical properties enabling formulation into a suitable form (e.g., tablet, parenteral solution) to enable adequate delivery of the drug to the site of action. Methods must be developed based on either chemical assay or bioassay to enable characterization of the pharmacodynamic and pharmacokinetic properties of the drug in man. Finally, there must exist defined and quantifiable measures of the non-disease-related effects of the drug; that is, we must be able to quantify the treatment-emergent adverse events associated with drug use in order to measure this component of the overall risk associated with use of the drug.

IV. ODDS OF SUCCESSFUL DRUG DEVELOPMENT

Let us presume that a drug can be successfully developed only if appropriate responses are available to each of the eight questions listed in Table 1. If each question has the bimodal outcomes "appropriate for successful drug development" versus "inappropriate for successful drug development," then the random chance of success is $(1/2)^8$ or $1/256$. Cato [3] estimated that 1 of every 10 compounds entering clinical development results in an approved NDA. Comparing this $1/10$ success rate with random chance of $1/256$, it appears that the pharmaceutical industry performs about 25 times better than random chance alone!

The odds of successful drug development can be expanded by considering the attrition rates for potential drugs in chemical synthesis and preclinical studies. Cato [3] estimated that to achieve 1 approved NDA you must have 10 compounds enter clinical development; these 10 compounds were selected from 1,000 compounds entering preclinical pharmacological and toxicological studies; and these 1,000 compounds were selected from 10,000 chemicals presented from synthesis or natural products. Each step is also time consuming since development of the average new chemical entity requires 0.5 years in chemical synthesis, 3.5 years in preclinical pharmacology and toxicology, 6.6 years in clinical development, and 2.7 years of NDA review time for an average total development time of 13.3 years [3].

V. CHOOSING NEW CHEMICAL ENTITIES FOR DEVELOPMENT IN THE RESEARCH-BASED PHARMACEUTICAL INDUSTRY

The goal of the research-based pharmaceutical industry must be to develop new drugs that comprise major advances for therapy of various diseases. In order to get a quantitative index of success in attaining this goal, we reviewed all new chemical entities approved by FDA during the decade of the 1980s. A total of 217 new chemical entities were approved by FDA from 1980-1989 (Table 3). Of these drugs, 28 drugs (13%) were classified by FDA as 1AA/1A drugs, i.e., drugs offering an important therapeutic gain, while 67 drugs (31%) were classified as 1B drugs (i.e., drugs offering modest therapeutic gain), and 122 drugs (56%) were classified as 1C drugs (i.e., drugs offering little or no therapeutic gain). Table 4 provides a listing of the 1A and 1B drugs approved during the 1980s. These data are fascinating since they show that during the decade of the 1980s over half of the newly approved new chemical entities offered little or no therapeutic gain, while only 13% of the newly approved drugs achieved the goal of providing an important therapeutic gain. While these proportions of approvals do not quantitatively reflect the exact proportions of resources (time, money, manpower) used in their discovery and development, they do provide a qualitative index of the relative resources invested in achieving important therapeutic gains. At any given time in the research-based pharmaceutical industry in the U.S., one may find approximately 10% of projects devoted to pioneer drugs promising important

Table 3. Number of new chemical entities approved by FDA in the decade of the 1980s [4-13].

Calendar Year	Number of NCEs Approved	FDA Therapeutic Rating		
		1A	1B	1C
1980	12	2	2	8
1981	27	2	11	14
1982	28	4	5	19
1983	14	4	1	9
1984	22	2	8	12
1985	30	3	15	12
1986	20	1	8	11
1987	21	2	5	14
1988	20	4	6	10
1989	23	4	6	13
TOTALS	217	28 (13%)	67 (31%)	122 (56%)

Table 4. List of new chemical entities (by year of approval) that attained a 1AA, 1A, or 1B therapeutic rating from FDA [4–13].

Year of Approval	Therapeutic Rating	Trade Name	Indication
1980	1-A	Ritodrine	smooth muscle relaxant
	1-A	Vansil	antischistosomal
	1-B	Viroptic	antiviral
	1-B	Zomax	anti-inflammatory
1981	1-A	Nizoral	systemic antifungal
	1-A	Prostin VR	ductus arteriosus in newborns
	1-B	Capoten	antihypertensive
	1-B	Carafate	antiulcer
	1-B	Claforan	antibacterial
	1-B	Fansidar	antimalarial
	1-B	Isoptin & Calan	antiarrhythmic
	1-B	Moxam	antibacterial
	1-B	Nasalide	allergic rhinitis
	1-B	Pipracil	antibacterial
	1-B	Procardia	antianginal
	1-B	Proventil	bronchodilator
	1-B	Secretin-Kabi	pancreatic diagnostic
1982	1A	Accutane	severe cystic acne
	1A	Biltricide	antischistosomal
	1A	Calcibind Phosphate	hypercalciurea type I with recurrent calcium nephrolithiasis
	1A	Chymodiactin	herniated disc
	1A	Niclocide	antihelminthic
	1B	Dolobid	anti-inflammatory, analgesic
	1B	Factrel	hormonal diagnostic
	1B	Hepatolite	diagnostic imaging
	1B	Zovirax	antiviral
1983	1A	Chenix	gallstone dissolution
	1A	Lithostat	decrease urinary ammonia and alkalinity
	1A	Sandimmune	immunosuppresant
	1A	VePesid	antineoplastic agent
	1B	Tracrium	neuromuscular blocker

Table 4 (*Continued*)

Year of Approval	Therapeutic Rating	Trade Name	Indication
1984	1A	Pentam 300	antiprotozoal agent
	1A	Trental	intermittent claudication
	1B	Augmentin 250	antibacterial/beta-lactamase inhibitor
	1B	Monocid	antibacterial
	1B	Nicorette	tobacco smoking withdrawal
	1B	Normodyne	antihypertensive
	1B	Rocephin	antibacterial
	1B	Sufenta	anesthetic/analgesic
	1B	Tonocard	anti-arrhythmic
	1B	Trexan	narcotic antagonist
1985	1A	Cordarone	anti-arrhythmic
	1A	Protropin	human growth hormone
	1A	Virazole	antiviral
	1B	Betoptic	glaucoma
	1B	L-Carnitine	carnitine deficiency
	1B	Cuprid	Wilson's disease
	1B	Fortaz	antibacterial
	1B	indium-111 oxyquinolone	diagnostic agent
	1B	Lupron	synthetic gonadotropin releasing hormone
	1B	Marinol	anti-emetic
	1B	Mexitil	anti-arrhythmic
	1B	Moctanin	gallstone dissolution
	1B	Primaxin	antibacterial
	1B	Ridaura	anti-arthritic
	1B	Seldane	antihistamine
	1B	Tambocor	anti-arrhythmic
	1B	Vasotec	antihypertensive
	1B	Wellbutrin	antidepressant

Table 4 (*Continued*)

Year of Approval	Therapeutic Rating	Trade Name	Indication
1986	1-A	Lamprene	leprosy
	1-B	Atrovent	COPD
	1-B	Azactam	antibacterial
	1-B	Brevibloc	beta-blocker
	1-B	Buspar	anxiolytic
	1-B	Cibacalcin	Paget's disease
	1-B	Enkaid	anti-arrhythmic
	1-B	Nix	pediculocide
	1-B	Noroxin	antibacterial
	1-B	Ocufen	inhibition of intraoperative miosis
	1-B	Provocholine	asthma diagnostic
	1-B	Tegison	antipsoriatic
1987	1-AA	Retrovir	HIV infection
	1-A	Mevacor	hypercholesterolemia
	1-B	Cipro	antibacterial
	1-B	Deursil	gallstone dissolution
	1-B	Prozac	antidepressant
	1-B	Rowasa	ulcerative colitis; proctosia moiditis; proctitis
	1-B	Ucephan	hyperammonemia due to urea cycle enzymopathies
1988	1-A	Cytotec	prevention of NSAID- induced ulcers
	1-A	Ifex	third-line chemotherapy of germ cell testicular cancer
	1-A	Nimotop	subarachnoid hemorrhage
	1-A	Sandostatin	carcinoid tumors and VIPomas
	1B	Ceretec	adjunct in detection of stroke
	1B	Ethamolin	prevention of rebleeding of esophageal varices
	1B	Magnevist	brain imaging agent

Table 4 (*Continued*)

Year of Approval	Therapeutic Rating	Trade Name	Indication
	1B	Mesnex	prevention of ifosfamide-induced hemorrhagic cystitis
	1B	Permax	adjunct to levodopa/ carbidopa for Parkinson's disease
1989	1AA	Cytovene	CMV retinitis in immunocompromised patients
	1A	Anafranil	obsessive compulsive disorder
	1A	Clozaril	second-line treatment of schizophrenia
	1A	Lariam	treatment and prophylaxis of malaria
	1B	Adenocard	paroxysmal supraventricular tachycardia
	1B	Eldepryl	adjunct to levodopa/ carbidopa in Parkinsonian patients
	1B	Eulexin	concomitant treatment with leuprolide for metastatic prostate cancer
	1B	Losec	GERD, erosive esophagitis, Zollinger-Ellison syndrome
	1B	Paraplatin	palliative treatment of recurrent ovarian cancer
	1B	Toradol	short-term management of pain

therapeutic gains, about 30% of resources devoted to non-pioneer projects promising some therapeutic gain, and over half the resources allocated to purely "me too" projects that promise little, if any, therapeutic gain. We will refer to these "me too" products as patented generic drugs. The corresponding profile of financial risks and potential returns is a topic discussed briefly in a later chapter of this book.

REFERENCES

1. Cohn JP. The beginnings: laboratory and animal studies. In: *From Test Tube to Patient: New Drug Development in the United States.* Special report by FDA Consumer. Rockville, MD: U.S. Food and Drug administration, January, 1988, pages 8–11.
2. Miller L, Dalton M, Vestal R, Perkins JG, Lyon G. Delays in the drug approval process: recent trends. *J. Clin. Res. Drug Development 2*: 31–45 (1988).
3. Cato AE. The challenge of the clinical development of drugs. In: *Clinical Drug Trials and Tribulations* (Cato AE, ed.). New York: Marcel Dekker, Inc., 1988, Chapter 1, pp. 1–16.
4. New chemical entities approved by FDA in 1981. *F-D-C Reports (The Pink Sheet)* 44: 17 (January 11, 1982).
5. FDA's 1982 new chemical entity approvals. *F-D-C Reports (The Pink Sheet)* 45: 4 (January 17, 1983).
6. FDA 1983 new chemical entity approvals. *F-D-C Reports (The Pink Sheet)* 46: 4 (January 16, 1984).
7. FDA 1984 new chemical entity approvals. *F-D-C Reports (The Pink Sheet)* 47: 6 (January 7, 1985).
8. FDA 1985 new chemical entity approvals. *F-D-C Reports (The Pink Sheet)* 48: 9 (January 13, 1986).
9. FDA's 1986 new molecular entity approvals. *F-D-C Reports (The Pink Sheet)* 49: 9 (January 5, 1987).
10. FDA's new molecular entity approvals. *F-D-C Reports (The Pink Sheet)* 50: 11 (January 11, 1988).
11. FDA's new molecular entity approvals. *F-D-C Reports (The Pink Sheet)* 51: 6 (January 9, 1989).
12. FDA's 1989 new molecular entity approvals. *F-D-C Reports (The Pink Sheet)* 52: 5 (January 8, 1990).
13. *New Drug Evaluation Statistical Report.* U.S. Department of Health and Human Services. April, 1987.

part two

Approaches to Clinical Drug Development

2
Purpose of Clinical Drug Development: Assessment of Benefits and Risks

A desire to take medicine is, perhaps,
the great feature which distinguishes
man from other animals.

Sir William Osler

I. INTRODUCTION

The process of developing investigational drugs is integrated traditionally into four overlapping phases. The goal of drug development is the introduction of new therapies to clinical medicine through benefit/risk assessment, i.e., the assessment of the benefits gained and the risks incurred in association with the new drug. Benefit assessment is unique to each individual disease setting in which the drug may comprise an effective treatment. In contrast, safety assessment is relatively standardized across many pharmacological classes of drugs. In this chapter, conventional approaches toward synthesis of a benefit/risk assessment from overall safety and efficacy data are discussed in the context of both major categories of disease and the clinical toxicities of drugs.

Formation of a benefit/risk assessment is more easily approached if we consider that investigational drugs are developed to provide benefit in three major disease categories: acute disease, episodic disease, and chronic disease. The nature of these three categories is described with specific examples of drug therapies in each category. Following elucidation of the disease-associated and drug-associated factors that determine the desired benefit and the acceptable risk, conventional approaches to benefit/risk assessment are described. Benefit assessment is the major focus of conventional methodologies.

II. BENEFIT/RISK ASSESSMENT

In the United States, the process of developing a chemical, from discovery to availability by prescription, involves the necessity for the developer to provide substantial evidence of its effectiveness and safety [1–4]. Evidence of effectiveness usually includes data to prove that the drug can eliminate or diminish the clinical consequences of some pathology better than placebo or at least as well as other therapies previously shown to be effective. Substantial evidence of safety consists predominantly of data collected in studies of patients with the diseases for which the drug may be indicated.

A benefit/risk assessment for a target patient population is formulated by integration of safety data and effectiveness data as required for new drug applications pursuant to the Federal Food, Drug, and Cosmetic Act [5]:

> Concisely compare kind and incidence of beneficial experience with kind and incidence of adverse experience found in clinical studies.

Formulation of an adequate benefit/risk assessment occurs in two stages. First, the epidemiology of the target disease and the toxicities of potential drug therapies must be considered together in order to form a general notion of acceptable risk in the specific therapeutic setting. Second, the appropriate data must be collected in well-designed, well-controlled clinical trials to enable evaluation of the actual benefits and risks associated with therapy and the disease.

The goal of the drug development process is introduction of new therapies to clinical medicine through evaluation of the benefit gained and the risks incurred as a result of therapy. This benefit/risk assessment enables characterization of the benefits and risks associated with therapy in light of the pathogenesis of a specific disease and, thereby, determines whether the benefits of therapy sufficiently outweigh the risks. Generally, the desired benefit is either known or easily identifiable based on the current understanding of the particular target disease [6]. Typically, the benefit consists of eliminating or reducing the adverse health consequences associated with the manifestations, unhindered progression, and sequelae of the disease. In this context, a pharmacologic effect of a given drug is not beneficial unless that effect explicitly reduces the manifestations or progression of a disease. Consequently, it is important to identify early in a drug discovery program the potential therapeutic benefits for various pharmacologically active entities. This may prove particularly relevant to the clinical development of agents whose receptor interactions are well understood in the absence of a defined relationship between the target receptors and the pathogenesis of any disease.

Construction of an adequate benefit/risk assessment must be founded on an understanding of the epidemiology of the disease to be treated and the desirable therapeutic benefit to be achieved. For purposes of drug development, we can consider three general classes of disease: (1) acute disease, i.e., disease occurring with a specific and continuous pathology during an isolated period of time and not commonly recurring spontaneously if cured (e.g., acute infectious disease such as uncomplicated gonorrhea); (2) episodic disease, i.e., disease characterized by recurrent acute manifestations, separated temporally by quiescent periods, as a result of the same or similar pathophysiology (e.g., ulcer disease, malaria, generalized seizure disorder); and (3) chronic disease, i.e., disease with continuous clinical manifestations due to irreversible pathological alteration of normal physiology such that the disease may be controllable, but not curable, by today's therapies (e.g., diabetes mellitus, hypertension). In each of these three categories, definition of the achievable benefit dictates the risks which are potentially acceptable for therapies.

A. Acute Disease

The adverse health consequences of an acute disease range from uncomfortable symptoms in the presence of largely normal function, as with the common cold, to death for diseases such as nosocomial bacterial pneumonia. Obviously, the goals of therapy are not the same at these extremes. For the relatively mild, self-limited, acute disease, paliation of the effects of the disease process is the desired benefit. Since the disease has minor, even trivial, short-term consequences, therapy-associated risks must also be trivial. Thus, the short-term risks must be reversible and relatively infrequent in their occurrence. Similarly, any therapy-associated long-term risk is unacceptable in this setting. As the degree of disease-associated adverse health consequences increases among the acute diseases, the benefit of reducing these consequences increases and thus the degree of tolerable therapy-associated risk increases. One example is the use of antibacterial agents in the treatment of acute bacterial infectious diseases. For example, bacterial meningitis in the pediatric patient may be immediately life-threatening and may be associated with long-term adverse neurological sequelae [7,8]. Consequently, rapid eradication of the infectious bacterium, defervescence, and ultimate cure without disease-related sequelae are the only beneficial responses that are totally acceptable. Attainment of this benefit often necessitates aggressive therapy (e.g.,intrathecal administration of an aminoglycoside plus one or more intravenous antibacterial drugs) with acceptance of higher therapy-associated risk. In this setting, transient subjective complaints or reversible major organ system dysfunctions may not preclude or even discourage the use of some antibacterial agents. In fact, antibacterial agents (e.g., chloramphenicol), which are known to produce irreversible major organ system damage in some patients, are used depending upon the gravity of the situation.

B. Episodic Disease

Episodic diseases are actually a series of acute disease episodes which recur periodically as a result of similar or related pathophysiology. Such diseases have both short-term risks during the acute episodes and long-term risks as a result of the recurrent nature of the disease. For example, the risk of a clinically significant or even life-threatening gastrointestinal hemorrhage in duodenal ulcer is relatively high during acute ulcerative episodes [9,10]. In the long-term, the risk of a recurrent hemorrhage is also present and may occur either from the previously healed lesion in 60–75% of patients [11,12] or from a different lesion in 20–30% of patients [12,13]. In addition, the scar tissue which may form after repeated cycles of ulceration and healing may cause stricture or complete obstruction. For an episodic disease, as for an acute disease, the desired therapeutic benefit must be specified in order to define the acceptable therapeutic risk. During the acute episodes, therapy must reduce the manifestations and promote normalization of the pathology of the disease. For ulcer disease, this means that therapy should render the patient asymptomatic and accelerate the re-epitheliazation process. In ulcer disease and other episodic diseases, transient subjective complaints are tolerable for therapy of acute episodes. However, therapy-associated major organ system dysfunctions, even if transient, are a cause of considerable concern since the therapeutic modality may be utilized repeatedly during a lifetime. Moreover, the acute therapies for episodic diseases should not increase the rate or severity of recurrence of the acute episodes. Thus, clinical trials on therapies for episodic disease must include characterization of the effect of investigational acute therapies on the long-term prognosis.

In view of the recurrent nature of episodic diseases, long-term management is of great concern due to the need to balance the risks of long-term therapy (either intermittent or continuous drug administration) against the benefits of controlling recurrent acute episodes of disease. One goal of long-term therapy must be to reduce the potential for disease-associated sequelae. This can be accomplished by rendering the acute episodes less severe (i.e., paliative treatment) and, in some cases, by actually reducing the number of occurrences of acute episodes (i.e., prophylaxis). If either paliation or prophylaxis are the objective of long-term therapy, the incidence of drug-induced organ dysfunctions must be rare. In addition, subjective complaints must be infrequent and mild so as not to discourage a patient from continuing long-term therapy.

Strategies for long-term therapeutic management in patients with various episodic diseases are somewhat controversial. Long-term management of ulcer disease provides a useful example. It has been debated whether continuous therapy or intermittent treatment of acute episodes of ulcer disease is the preferred strategy for long-term management [14–16]. These controversies can best be resolved for each individual patient based on consideration of their own benefit/risk profile. Patients with high disease-associated risk from the recurrent acute episodes of the disease are candidates for continuous therapy. Intermittent therapy of acute episodes is the preferred strategy when the continuous therapy strategy incurs long-term therapy-associated risk unacceptable to a patient. The latter may occur, for example, in a patient whose episodic disease is not the disease responsible for his greatest morbidity or risk of mortality. Clinical trials must evaluate a broad range of patients in order to identify those patient subgroups which are most in need of either continuous or intermittent therapy for their episodic disease. One method which may prove useful in identifying the patient subgroups amenable to different therapies is randomized evaluation of different therapies in an individual patient, i.e., the so-called "n of 1" study [17]. Other creative strategies for systematic therapeutic optimization in the individual patient with an episodic disease must be developed.

C. Chronic Disease

Chronic diseases are the result of persistent and pathological alterations of normal physiology. Such diseases may be controllable, but not curable, by today's therapies. The disease risks are generally only long term, that is, the increased morbidity and mortality associated with the disease are generally only evident after prolonged presence of the disease. For example, the renal damage or left ventricular hypertrophy associated with essential hypertension and the crippling associated with rheumatoid arthritis are long-term manifestations of these respective diseases. For these and other chronic diseases, the immediate goal of therapy is control, i.e., therapeutic stabilization of the pathophysiology associated with the disease and maintenance of that stabilized state. The result of such control should be decreased morbidity or decreased mortality or decreases in both morbidity and mortality. By controlling the disease process, the morbidity associated with the disease will not progress. It is also desirable to reduce some of the short-term morbid manifestations of chronic diseases. However, improvement in the disease manifestations does not constitute a cure of the underlying disease. For example, some studies suggest that disease-modifying anti-rheumatic drugs (DMARDs) can slow the degenerative process associated with rheumatoid arthritis, but they do not remove the pathophysiology of rheumatoid arthritis [18–23]. The patient with arthritis who is at some point left untreated will generally within a few months suffer recurrence of the disease manifestations which were reduced or absent during DMARD therapy [23].

The persistent pathophysiology of chronic diseases is of major importance in discerning the acceptable risks of therapy. While paliative management of immediate symptoms is necessary, the ultimate desired therapeutic benefit in chronic diseases can only be discussed in terms of reduction of long-term morbidity and mortality. For example, one goal of drug therapy of congestive heart failure is to increase functionality for considerable periods of time (i.e., months to years) and thereby decrease morbidity. For the patient who may only benefit from drug therapy for a short time (i.e., days to weeks), alternative therapies such as heart transplant may be considered. In view of the necessity to administer continuous drug therapy for very long periods of time (i.e., decades) for a chronic disease, substantial therapy-associated short-term risk is unacceptable. Subjective complaints are tolerable as short-term risks if they do not deter continuation of therapy. Alterations in major organ function must be either beneficial, trivial, or reversible. Virtually any short-term, irreversible, major organ system toxicity renders use of the drug an unacceptable risk. Long-term therapy-associated risks are similarly intolerable. Most chronic diseases are either life-threatening or disabling only in the long term. Any therapy that might add to these long-term disease-associated hazards would be undesirable.

One example of this compounded long-term hazard comes from therapy of mild hypertension. Diuretic therapy has been reported to increase the incidence of cardiac arrhythmias, possibly secondary to hypokalemia [24–33]. Such arrhythmogenic effects may make certain diuretics have an unacceptable benefit/risk profile for long-term treatment. Potassium supplementation can mitigate the arrhythmogenic effects of some diuretics [34].

The importance of evaluating risks associated with long-term therapy will be illustrated further by brief discussion of some of the controversies involved in the therapies of three chronic diseases, i.e., hypertension, congestive heart failure, and rheumatoid arthritis.

1. Hypertension

For years, it has been well accepted that the pharmacological treatment of patients with elevated blood pressure was beneficial. Patients with diastolic blood pressures averaging 105 mm Hg and above were found to have high hypertension-associated risk and antihypertensive therapy supplied a significant benefit in terms of associated reduction in morbidity and mortality [35–37]. More recently, considerable attention has been focused on the treatment of patients with lesser blood pressure elevations. Several epidemiological studies have been conducted throughout the world to evaluate the benefits of therapies in patients with diastolic blood pressure between 90 and 109 mm Hg [35,36,38–46]. These clinical studies have been the subject of a large number of papers and differing views. At present, it appears that the data are, at best, equivocal. From a population point of view, the benefit of the reduced cardiac mortality in this group of mildly hypertensive patients is quite small, i.e., on the order of two to seven patients per thousand patient years [40,41,43]. However, the risk of therapy is not trivial since, for example, approximately 15% of patients were discontinued from the Medical Research Council trial due to adverse events experienced while on therapy (i.e., thiazide diuretic or propranolol). Such an incidence of discontinuation of therapy due to adverse events is not atypical of incidences reported in controlled trials for various drug therapies used for other chronic diseases. In some studies in hypertensive patients, selected therapies have been associated with an increase in time lost from work [47], impotence [48], and a variety of other effects indicative of diminished quality of life [49]. Some studies have suggested that diuretics, traditional first-line agents in the treatment of hypertension, may predispose some patients to more frequent ventricular premature contractions [25,26]. Thus, application of benefit/risk principles makes it preferable to identify individual patients or patient types with benefit/risk profiles amenable to maintenance drug therapy, rather than treating large populations of people without substantial evidence of global benefit [50–52]. In this regard, elevated blood pressure readings provide necessary, but not sufficient, evidence to identify patients with both mild hypertension and its disease-associated risks. Some researchers have attempted to identify some "marker" for the disease of hypertension as an aid to screening for the disease [53–58]. The Framingham Study provided evidence of lifestyle characteristics associated with hypertension-related risk [59,60]. While these efforts may lead to better ways to identify therapy-requiring mildly hypertensive patients in the future, use of increased caution prior to initiation of drug therapy for patients with mild hypertension may become more acceptable in view of emerging evidence of the long-term benefit of non-pharmacological approaches to initial therapeutic management (i.e., weight loss, restriction of salt intake, restriction of ethanol intake, and cessation of smoking) [61,62] and the high placebo response rate in the Australian trial [43,63].

2. Congestive Heart Failure

No therapy has been clearly demonstrated to increase life expectancy of patients with congestive heart failure [64–67]. In fact, the efficacy and safety of the traditional therapies of diuretics and digitalis glycosides are now controversial [68–71]. Some of the currently available drugs diminish morbidity by objective improvement in cardiac performance or increases in functionality and exercise tolerance. These effects are observed with both inotropic agents and vasodilator therapy [72–75]. However, these therapeutic modalities have clear and different risks. Thus, balancing the benefits of therapies that have not been shown to reduce mortality and the drug-associated risks (e.g., sudden cardiac death at one extreme [76,77]) has presented a challenge in benefit/risk assessment.

3. Rheumatoid Arthritis

Rheumatoid arthritis is a chronic disease providing an opportunity to compare two therapeutic approaches with different benefit/risk profiles as a result of their different therapeutic effects. The non-steroidal anti-inflammatory drugs (NSAIDs) can reduce morbidity without altering disease progression. NSAIDs have been administered for paliation by short-term, "intermittent prn," and long-term continuous regimens. In contrast, some work suggests that DMARDs can slow degeneration of bone in order to provide remission and a reduction in morbidity. Since the DMARDs will not eradicate the arthritic pathophysiology, a strategy of continuous use or long-term intermittent use is appropriate. Clearly, the comparative toxicities of long-term use of both of these drug classes, some of which might be tolerable in an acute therapy situation, are an important consideration to the comparative benefit/risk assessment of these drugs in the arthritic patient.

III. APPROACHES TO BENEFIT/RISK ASSESSMENT

We have described three general categories of disease which comprise settings for evaluation of benefits and risks. The process of assessing benefits is highly variable since the specific therapeutic benefits are dictated by the unique characteristics of the disease to be treated. In contrast, the process of assessing the risks associated with investigational drugs is at present quite uniform across many drug classes and diseases.

The safety and efficacy of investigational drugs is commonly assessed as a composite of clinical data and laboratory data in both the healthy volunteers or patient volunteers enrolled in Phase I trials and the target patient population in Phase II and III trials. Table 1 summarizes the principal goals of the four phases of drug development. Across Phases I–III, the primary objective of benefit assessment is to quantify the relationship between dose and parameters of therapeutic effect, while the primary objective of safety assessment is to quantitatively characterize the relationship to dose of the frequencies and severities of adverse events. Therefore, conduct of Phases I–III is an exercise in elucidation of the comparative dose-therapeutic response and dose-toxic effect profiles. This focus of the clinical drug development process will be explored in detail in Chapter 4.

Prior to initial clinical trials, the potential major organ system toxicity of a new compound and the routes of elimination of the compound can be studied in part through use of animal models in which major organ system function is radically diminished by either chemical or surgical methods (Table 2). The new drug is then administered to these animals and they are monitored for changes in both objective and subjective parameters. Specimens of biological fluids (e.g., blood, urine) may be collected to characterize disposition of the drug. While such studies may be of some use, they are limited by the technical difficulties in creating some of these models (e.g., portacaval shunt rat), the high intrinsic variability in the degree of functional impairment produced by the various experimental methods, and the failure of these models to mimic any stable level of steady-state, impaired, organ function. Thus, animal models do provide some useful early information, but drug-induced illnesses must also be evaluated in humans with some major organ dysfunctions.

A. Methods of Clinical Safety Assessment

Clinical safety data consists of the results of serial physical examinations and evaluation of clinical adverse events. The following six different methods are used to evaluate clinical adverse events:

1. Observation of adverse events by a trained investigator
2. Recording of adverse events reported spontaneously by the patient
3. Patient diary card
4. Assessment of events reported by the patient in response to a verbal probe using a standard question (e.g., "How do you feel?")
5. Patient self-assessment checklist
6. Physician-administered questionnaire

Table 1. Principal goals of each phase of clinical drug development.

Phase	Typical Population	Safety Assessment Goal	Efficacy Assessment Goal	Other Goals
I	Healthy volunteers and patient volunteers	Single-Dose Studies: (1) identify the maximum "no effect" dose (2) identify the threshold toxic dose (3) identify the maximum tolerated dose (4) develop single dose-toxic effect relationships Multiple-Dose Studies: (1) identify the maximum "no effect" dosage regimen (2) identify the threshold toxic dosage regimen (3) identify the maximum tolerated dosage regimen (4) develop multiple dose-toxic effect relationships (5) estimate range of tolerated doses for exploration in Phase II	Single-Dose Studies: (1) identify and measure laboratory and clinical predictive correlates of efficacy between volunteers and the target patient population Multiple-Dose Studies: (1) measure laboratory and clinical predictive correlates of efficacy between volunteers and the target patient population	(1) pharmacokinetic characterization (including mass balance) (2) identification of drug metabolites (1) characterization of steady-state pharmacokinetic properties (including mass balance) and pharmacodynamic properties (2) identification of drug metabolites
II	Selected patient population (low heterogeneity)	(1) identify the maximum "no effect" dosage regimen (2) identify the threshold toxic dosage regimen	(1) demonstrate presence or absence of any degree of efficacy at any dosage regimen (2) demonstrate presence or	(1) pharmacokinetic characterization in patients (2) explore relationship between

	(3) identify the maximum tolerated dosage regimen (4) identify the plateau dose (5) characterize dose-toxic effect relationships (6) identify any high-incidence toxicities (catastrophic and non-catastrophic)	absence of any degree of efficacy at a safe dosage regimen (3) characterize dose-therapeutic effect relationships (4) conduct initial adequate and well-controlled efficacy trials	pharmacokinetic properties and pharmacological effects of the drug (3) test potential laboratory predictors of efficacy and safety
III Target patient poulation (moderate heterogeneity)	(1) further identify and characterize catastrophic toxicities (2) identify non-catastrophic toxicities and quantify their incidence (3) as appropriate, initiate long-term safety monitoring for patients on chronic medication	(1) expanded adequate and well-controlled efficacy trials (2) pilot efficacy studies in expanded indication areas to be developed in supplements	(1) studies to provide efficacy data needed largely to support competitive marketing of the drug (2) larger scale characterization of relationship between pharmacokinetic properties and pharmacological effects
IV General medical population (high heterogeneity)	(1) post-marketing safety monitoring in clinical trials (2) comparative safety trials needed for competitive marketing (3) identify lower incidence catastrophic toxicities (4) identify patient sub-populations at high risk of adverse events	(1) expanded efficacy studies in promising areas identified in pilot studies (2) comparative efficacy trials needed for competitive marketing	

Table 2. Some animal models of renal insufficiency and hepatic insufficiency.

Model	Animal Species	Method
Renal Insufficiency	rat	uranyl nitrate injection [78–81]
		bilateral ureteral ligation [80–81]
		one-stage five-sixths nephrectomy [81]
		two-stage five-sixths nephrectomy [81]
Hepatic Insufficiency	rat	two-thirds hepatectomy [82,83]
	rat	two-stage hepatectomy [84]
	dog	three-stage hepatectomy [85]
	rat	exclusionary hepatectomy [86]
	rat	portal-systemic shunt [87,88]
	cat	portal-systemic shunt [89]
	dog	portal-systemic shunt [81,90]
	rat, dog	carbon tetrachloride [91–93]
	rat	alpha-naphthylisothiocyanate [94]

The comparative advantages and disadvantages of each of these six methods are listed in Table 3. While it is clear that these methods produce quantitatively different information, the qualitative differences in their results have not been extensively evaluated in controlled trials. The verbal probe method is widely used in both comparative and non-comparative studies as a means to detect both adverse events which are predictable for the drug class and unpredictable events which may be previously undiscovered for the investigational drug. Table 4 catalogs some standard questions that have been used as verbal probes in clinical trials.

Self-assessment checklists and physician-administered questionnaires are used almost exclusively in comparative clinical studies in an effort to quantify the comparative incidences of predictable adverse events for members of a given drug class in comparison to an active control or placebo. One of these latter two methods is commonly used in combination with the verbal probe method in comparative clinical trials for a new drug. These approaches are usually supplemented with recording all spontaneous reports from the patient. The other methods listed in Table 3 are not commonly used due to the excessive time required for "observation by the investigator" and the large amount of unstructured information elicited by patient diary cards. Only with great effort can such unstructured information be interpreted, reduced using a standard adverse event dictionary, and summarized.

In addition to these approaches to monitoring specific adverse events, the impact of investigational drugs administered continuously for episodic or chronic diseases on functionality and the quality of life of patients should be assessed [122–124]. Such quality of life assessments have been done for antihypertensive drugs [125,126], various surgical procedures [127–132], cancer interventions [133,134], cardiac disease therapy [135,136], and antirheumatic therapy [137]. If these data are obtained during the drug development process, they could be uniquely useful to physicians' efforts to choose between intermittent and continuous therapy for a patient with an episodic disease, as well as choices among alternative therapies for a patient with a chronic disease.

B. Methods of Laboratory Safety Assessment

Laboratory safety data are gathered by serial determinations of selected clinical laboratory tests before initiating therapy with the study drug, periodically during therapy with the study drug, and periodically after discontinuation of treatment with the study drug. Data must be collected in order to assess the drug's effects on laboratory indices of hematopoietic, hepatic, and renal functions. The presence of potentially drug-related changes is commonly assessed by comparing intra-treatment and post-treatment test results with pre-treatment test results for a battery of blood chemistry, hematology, and urinalysis tests.

For some drugs, additional safety data must be obtained using a variety of procedures to assess cardiac, auditory, ophthalmic, and metabolic functions. Clinical tests such as the electrocardiogram, ophthalmological testing (e.g., tonometry, fundoscopy, visual field testing), audiometric testing, and specialty renal function tests must be conducted as indicated by the pharmacological properties of the specific investigational drug. The specific laboratory tests conducted and examples of the types of drug-related effects that each test may detect have been presented in summary form previously [138].

IV. SUMMARY OF CURRENT APPROACHES

In the context of benefit/risk assessment as described above, the intentions of new drug development can be detailed. For the individual patient, disease may be cured or controlled through optimal clinical use of pharmacological entities. Optimal clinical use affords maximum benefit with minimum risk associated with drug-related toxicities. The nature of classical dose-response relationships dictates our desire to discover therapies with an acceptable magnitude of separation between the doses associated with beneficial effects on the disease process and the doses associated with unacceptable adverse medical events. Substantial experimental evidence of the clinical efficacy and safety of the new drug must be

Table 3. Comparative advantages and disadvantages of methods of assessing clinical adverse events.

Method	Advantages	Disadvantages
Observation by Investigator	1. "leading" the patient is unlikely 2. does not require patient literacy (e.g., useful in children, illiterate adults) 3. focused on detecting objective events	1. may be inadequate incentive for patient to volunteer information 2. inadequate detection of subjective events 3. requires time of investigator for intensive observation
Spontaneous Reporting	1. "leading" the patient is unlikely 2. no pressure on patient to report 3. does not require patient literacy (e.g., useful in children, illiterate adults) 4. capable of detecting both predictable (i.e., drug class) and unpredictable events	1. requires patient initiative to make the report 2. does not assure that staff see the patient regularly regarding adverse events 3. requires patient description of information to be reported
Patient Diary Card [95–97]	1. patient uses his own words to describe events ("leading" the patient is unlikely) 2. capable of detecting both predictable (i.e., drug class) and unpredictable events	1. tends to elicit a large amount of unstructured information 2. patient may under-report or over-report events 3. diary cards can be lost 4. requires literate patients 5. patient may feel obliged to report something 6. does not assure conversations with the patient
Verbal Probe via Standard Question [95,98–103]	1. "leading" the patient is unlikely 2. presents specific opportunities for patients to provide data with minimal initiative 3. may facilitate conversation and rapport with patient 4. does not require literacy 5. useful in both controlled and uncontrolled trials 6. may be used in addition to self-assessment checklist or physician-administered question 7. capable of detecting both predictable (i.e., drug class) and unpredictable events	1. patient may feel obliged to report something 2. requires patient to initially decide what must be reported, depending on phrasing of the question 3. may elicit less information than checklists on potentially embarrassing events (e.g., sexual dysfunction)

Self-Assessment Checklist [95,97,99,100,104–107]

1. patient does not differentiate reportable events
2. requires little patient initiative
3. items can be varied by drug class, sex of patient, or other variables
4. collects more accurate data about potentially embarrassing events (e.g., sexual dysfunction)
5. tends to result in higher incidence of drug-related events than verbal probe
6. allows self-rating of severity as mild/moderate/severe or on a visual analogue scale
7. requires little time of investigator to administer
8. tends to result in more ratings of higher severity than verbal probe

1. "leading" the patient is more likely; items have to be worded carefully
2. patient may feel obliged to report something
3. does not assure conversations with patient
4. requires literate patients
5. detects only predictable (i.e., drug class) events
6. not useful in uncontrolled trials

Physician-Administered Questionnaire [95,98,101,118–120]

1. patient does not differentiate reportable events from non-reportable events
2. requires little patient initiative
3. assures conversation between investigator and patient
4. does not require literacy (e.g., useful in children, illiterate adults)
5. questions can be varied by drug class, sex of patient, age of patient, or other variables
6. tends to result in higher incidence of drug-related events than verbal probe
7. tends to result in more ratings of higher severity than verbal probe

1. needs great care in wording questions
2. patient may feel obliged to report something
3. requires time from investigator to administer
4. detects only predictable (i.e., drug class) events
5. presents a more limited list of questions than checklists since this requires physician time for administration
6. may collect less accurate data on potentially embarrassing events (e.g., sexual dysfunction)
7. not useful in uncontrolled trials
8. may obscure important side effects among trivial complaints

Table 4. Standard questions used for verbal probe in clinical trials.

Verbal Probe	Drugs Studied
1. "Have you noticed any change in bodily function or had any physical complaints in the past week?" [98]	chlorpromazine
2. "How are you feeling?" then, "How else are you feeling?" then, "How does the drug make you feel?" [95]	amitriptyline, iprindole, diazepam, chlordiazepoxide, fluphenazine
3. "Have you noticed any new symptoms which might be related to the treatment?" [100]	aspirin or fenoprofen
4. "Have you had any medical problems since your last visit?" [101]	mesoridazine
5. "Any problems?" [102]	labetalol
6. "Did you experience any unpleasant effects from the medicine you took?" [103]	none
7. "Have you felt different in any way since your last visit?" [121]	none

collected by the investigators and sponsor. The Federal Food Drug and Cosmetic Act states [139]:

> Such persons shall submit to the Secretary as a part of application (1) full reports of investigations which have been made to show whether or not such drug is safe for use and whether such drug is effective in use;

The dogmatic language of this statement suggests that safety and efficacy are absolute entities. However, benefit/risk assessment is an exercise in optimization. This optimization process is a joint effort of the drug developer, investigators, patients, and the FDA. The information presented in this chapter suggests that the current benefit/risk assessment process is not optimal. The reasons for sub-optimal approaches to benefit/risk assessment are the subject of the next chapter.

REFERENCES

1. Barron BA, Bukantz SC. The evaluation of new drugs: current Food and Drug Administration regulations and statistical aspects of clinical trials. *Arch. Intern. Med. 119*: 547–556 (1967).

2. Hamner CE (ed.). *Drug Development.* Boca Raton, FL: CRC Press, Inc.; 1982.

3. Nwangwu PU (ed.). *Concepts and Strategies in New Drug Development.* New York: Praeger Publishers; 1983.

4. Matoren GM (ed.). *The Clinical Research Process in the Pharmaceutical Industry.* New York: Marcel Dekker Inc.; 1984.

5. Title 21, Code of Federal Regulations, article 314.1. Washington, D.C.: U.S. Government Printing Office, 1980, page 94.

6. Fries JF, Ehrlich GE. *Prognosis. Contemporary Outcomes of Disease.* Bowie, MD: Charles Press Publishers; 1981.

7. Sell SHW, Webb WW, Pate JE, Doyne EO. Psychological sequelae of bacterial meningitis: two controlled studies. *Pediatrics 49:* 212–217 (1972).

8. Menkes JH. Improving the long-term outlook in bacterial meningitis. *Lancet 2:* 559–560 (1979).

9. Silverstein FE, Gilbert DA, Tedesco FJ, Buenger NK, Persing J. The National ASGE survey on upper gastrointestinal bleeding. II. Clinical prognostic factors. *Gastrointest. Endosc. 27:* 80–93 (1981).

10. Larson DE, Farnell MB. Upper gastrointestinal hemorrhage. *Mayo Clin. Proc. 58:* 371–387 (1983).

11. Palmer ED. The vigorous diagnostic approach to upper gastrointestinal tract hemorrhage. A 23 year prospective study of 14,000 patients. *JAMA 207:* 1477–1480 (1969).

12. Cotton PB, Rosenberg MT, Waldram RP, Axon AT. Early endoscopy of oesophagus, stomach, and duodenal bulb in patients with hematemesis and melaena. *Brit. Med. J. 2:* 505–509 (1973).

13. Katon RM, Smith FW. Panendoscopy in the early diagnosis of acute upper gastrointestinal bleeding. *Gastroenterology 65:* 728–734 (1973).

14. Pounder RE. Approaches to the long-term treatment of duodenal ulceration. In: Misiewicz JJ, Wood JR, eds. *Ranitidine Therapeutic Advances.* Amsterdam: Excerpta Medica, Chapter 1, 1984: 1–13.

15. Robinson M. Review of peptic ulcer maintenance trials. *Amer. J. Med. 77* (Suppl. 5B): 23–29 (1984).

16. Van Deventer DM. Approaches to the long-term treatment of duodenal ulcer disease. *Amer. J. Med. 77* (Suppl. 5B): 15–22 (1984).

17. Guyatt G, Sackett D, Taylor DW, Chong J, Roberts R, Pugsley S. Determining optimal therapy - randomized trials in individual patients. *N. Engl. J. Med. 314:* 889–892 (1986).

18. Constable TJ, Crockson RA, Crockson AP, McConkey B. Drug treatment of rheumatoid arthritis. *Lancet 1:* 1176–1180 (1975).

19. Wright V, Amos R. Do drugs change the course of rheumatoid arthritis? *Brit. Med. J. 280:* 964–966 (1980).

20. Iannuzzi L, Dawson N, Zein N, Kushner I. Does drug therapy slow radiographic deterioration in rheumatoid arthritis? *New Engl. J. Med. 309:* 1023–1028 (1983).

21. Lipsky PE. Remission-inducing therapy in rheumatoid arthritis. *Amer. J. Med. 75*: 40–49 (1983).
22. Pinals RS. Approaches to rheumatoid arthritis and osteoarthritis: an overview. *Amer. J. Med. 75*: 2–9 (1983).
23. O'Duffy JD, Luthra HS. Current status of disease- modifying drugs in progressive rheumatoid arthritis. *Drugs 27*: 373–377 (1984).
24. McMahon FG. Thiazides. In: *Management of Essential Hypertension.* Mount Kisco, N.Y.: Futura Publishing Co., Inc., Chapter 2, 1978: 21–54.
25. Hollifield JW, Slaton PE. Thiazide diuretics, hypokalemia and cardiac arrhythmias. *Acta Medica Scandinavica 647* (Suppl.): 67–73 (1981).
26. Holland OB, Nixon JV, Kuhnert L. Diuretic-induced ventricular ectopic activity. *Amer. J. Med. 70*: 762–768 (1981).
27. Harrington JT, Isner JM, Kassirer JP. Our national obsession with potassium. *Amer. J. Med. 73*: 155–159 (1982).
28. Medical Research Council Working Party on Mild to Moderate Hypertension. Ventricular extrasystoles during thiazide treatment: substudy of MRC mild hypertension trial. *Brit. Med. J. 287*: 1249–1253 (1983).
29. Struthers AD, Whitesmith R, Reid JL. Prior thiazide diuretic treatment increases adrenaline-induced hypokalemia. *Lancet 1*: 1358–1361 (1983).
30. Holland OB. The case for routinely normalizing serum potassium. In: Narins RG, ed. *Controversies in Nephrology and Hypertension.* New York: Churchill Livingstone; 1984: 345–358.
31. Holland OB. Diuretic-induced hypokalemia and ventricular arrhythmias. *Drugs 28* (Suppl. 1): 86–92 (1984).
32. Whelton PK. Diuretics and arrhythmias in the Medical Research Council trial. *Drugs 28* (Suppl. 1): 54–65 (1984).
33. Freis ED, Papademetriou V. How dangerous are diuretics? *Drugs 30*: 469–474 (1985).
34. Kassirer JP, Harrington JT. Diuretics and potassium metabolism: a reassessment of the need, effectiveness and safety of potassium therapy. *Kidney Int. 11*: 505–515 (1977).
35. Veterans Administration Cooperative Study Group on Antihypertensive Agents. Effects of treatment on morbidity in hypertension. Results in patients with diastolic blood pressures averaging 115–129 mm Hg. *JAMA 202*: 1028–1034 (1967).
36. Veterans Administration Cooperative Study Group on Antihypertensive Agents. Effects of treatment on morbidity in hypertension. II. Results in patients with diastolic blood pressure averaging 90 through 114 mm Hg. *JAMA 213*: 1143–1152 (1970).
37. Veterans Administration Cooperative Study Group on Antihypertensive Agents. Effects of treatment on morbidity and mortality. III. Influence of age, diastolic pressure, and prior cardiovascular disease; further analysis of side effects. *Circulation 45*: 991–1004 (1972).
38. Hypertension Detection and Follow-Up Program Cooperative Group. The hypertension detection and follow-up program. *Preventive Medicine 5*: 207–215 (1976).

39. Hypertension Detection and Follow-up Program Cooperative Group. Therapeutic control of blood pressure in the hypertension detection and follow-up program. *Preventive Medicine 8*: 2–13 (1979).

40. Hypertension Detection and Follow-up Program Cooperative Group. Five-year findings of the hypertension detection and follow-up program. I. Reduction in mortality of persons with high blood pressure, including mild hypertension. *JAMA 242*: 2562–2571 (1979).

41. Hypertension Detection and Follow-up Program Cooperative Group. The effect of treatment on mortality in "mild" hypertension. Results of the hypertension detection and follow-up program. *N. Engl. J. Med. 307*: 976–980 (1982).

42. Helgeland A. Treatment of mild hypertension: a five-year controlled drug trial. The Oslo study. *Amer. J. Med. 69*: 725–732 (1980).

43. Management Committee. The Australian therapeutic trial in mild hypertension. *Lancet 1*: 1261–1267 (1980).

44. Trafford JAP, Horn CR, O'Neal H, McGonigle R, Halford-Maw L, Evans R. Five-year follow-up of effects of treatment of mild and moderate hypertension. *Brit. Med. J. 282*: 1111–1113 (1981).

45. Amery A, Birkenhager W, Brixko P, et al. Mortality and morbidity results from the European Working Party on High Blood Pressure in the Elderly trial. *Lancet 1*: 1349–1354 (1985).

46. Medical Research Council Working Party. MRC trial of treatment of mild hypertension: principal results. *Brit. Med. J. 291*: 97–104 (1985).

47. Haynes RB, Sackett DL, Taylor GW, Gibson ES, Johnson AL. Absenteeism from work after detection and labeling of hypertensive patients. *N. Engl. J. Med. 299*: 741–744 (1978).

48. Report of Medical Research Council Working Party on mild to moderate hypertension. Adverse reactions to bendrofluazide and propranolol for the treatment of mild hypertension. *Lancet 2*: 539–543 (1981).

49. Dollery CT. Does it matter how blood pressure is reduced? *Clinical Science 61*: 413S–420S (1981).

50. Freis ED. Should mild hypertension be treated? *N. Engl. J. Med. 307*: 306–309 (1982).

51. Moser M, Gifford RW. Why less severe degrees of hypertension should be treated. *J. Hypertension 3*: 437–447 (1985).

52. Ramsey LE. Mild hypertension: treat patients, not populations. *J. Hypertension 3*: 449–455 (1985).

53. Swales JD. The hunt for renal hypertension. *Lancet 1*: 577–579 (1976).

54. Garay RP, Meyer P. A new test showing abnormal net Na+ and K+ fluxes in erythrocytes of essential hypertensive patients. *Lancet 1*: 349–353 (1979).

55. Garay RP, Dagher G, Pernollet MG, Devynck MA, Meyer P. Inherited defect in a Na+, K+-co-transport system in erythrocytes from essential hypertension patients. *Nature 284*: 281–283 (1980).

56. Nardi R, Sawa H, Carretta R, Bianchi M, Fernandes M. Characteristic variation in electrophoretic pattern of plasma proteins in essential hypertension. *Lancet 2*: 182–183 (1980).

57. Meyer P, Garay RP, Nazaret C, Dagher G, Bellet M, Broyer M, Feingold J. Inheritance of abnormal erythrocyte cation transport in essential hypertension. *Brit. Med. J. 282*: 1114–1117 (1981).

58. Poston L, Sewell RB, Wilkinson SP, Richardson PJ, Williams R, Clarkson EM, MacGregor GA, deWardener HE. Evidence for a circulating sodium transport inhibitor in essential hypertension. *Brit. Med. J. 282*: 847–849 (1981).

59. Kannel WB, Gordon T. Evaluation of cardiovascular risk in the elderly: the Framingham study. *Bull. N.Y. Acad. Med. 54*: 573–591 (1978).

60. Kannel WB, Sorlie P, McNamara PM. Prognosis after initial myocardial infarction: the Framingham Study. *Amer. J. Cardiol. 44*: 53–59 (1979).

61. Blaufoz MD, Langford HG, Oberman A, Hawkins CM, Wasserthiel-Smoller S, Cutter GR. Effect of dietary change on the return of hypertension after withdrawal of prolonged antihypertensive therapy (DISH). *J. Hypertension 2* (Suppl. 3): 179–181 (1984).

62. Stamler R, Stamler J, Grimm R, Gosch F, Dyer A, Berman R, Civinelli J, Elmer P, Fishman J, Van Heel N, McDonald A, McKeever P. Trial on control of hypertension by nutritional means: three-year results. *J. Hypertension 2* (Suppl. 3): 167–170 (1984).

63. Management Committee. Untreated mild hypertension. A report by the management committee of the Australian Therapeutic Trial in Mild Hypertension. *Lancet 1*: 185–191 (1982).

64. Franciosa JA, Wilen M, Ziesche S, Cohn J. Survival in men with with severe chronic left ventricular failure due to either coronary heart disease or idiopathic dilated cardiomyopathy. *Amer. J. Cardiol. 51*: 831–836 (1983).

65. Taylor SH, Storstein L. Diuretics and digitalis in the treatment of chronic heart failure. *Europ. Heart J. 4* (Suppl. A): 153–159 (1983).

66. Braunwald E, Colucci WS. Vasodilator therapy of heart failure. Has the promissory note been paid? *N. Engl. J. Med. 310*: 459–461 (1984).

67. Furberg CD, Yusuf S. Effect of vasodilators on survival in chronic congestive heart failure. *Amer. J. Cardiol. 55*: 1110–1112 (1985).

68. Moss AJ, Davis HT, Conrad DL, DeCamilla JJ, Odoroff CL. Digitalis associated cardiac mortality after myocardial infarction. *Circulation 64*: 1150–1156 (1981).

69. Chia-Sen Lee D, Johnson RA, Bingham JB, Leahy M, Dinsmore RE, Goroll AH, Newell JB, Strauss W, Haber E. Heart failure in outpatients. A randomized trial of digoxin versus placebo. *N. Engl. J. Med. 306*: 699–705 (1982).

70. Fleg JL, Gottlieb SH, Lakatta EG. Is digoxin really important in treatment of compensated heart failure? *Amer. J. Med. 73*: 244–250 (1982).

71. Ryan TJ, Bailey KR, McCabe CH, Luk S, Fisher LD, Mock MB, Killip T. The effect of digitalis on survival in high-risk patients with coronary artery disease (CASS). *Circulation 67*: 735–742 (1983).

72. Greenberg BH, Massie BM. Beneficial effects of afterload reduction therapy in patients with congestive heart failure and moderate aortic stenosis. *Circulation 61*: 1212–1216 (1980).

73. Massie B, Ports T, Chatterjee K, Parmley W, Ostland J, O'Young J, Haughom F. Long-term vasodilator therapy for heart failure: clinical response and its relationship to hemodynamic measurements. *Circulation 63*: 269–278 (1981).

74. Chatterjee K, Parmley WW. Vasodilator therapy for acute myocardial infarction and chronic congestive heart failure. *J. Amer. Coll. Cardiol. 1*: 133–153 (1983).

75. Schwartz AB, Chatterjee K. Vasodilator therapy in chronic congestive heart failure. *Drugs 26*: 148–173 (1983).

76. Shand DG, Pritchett ELC, Hammill SC, Stargel WW, Wagner GS. Pharmacokinetic studies: their role in determining therapeutic efficacy of agents designed to prevent sudden death. *Ann. N.Y. Acad. Sci. 382*: 238–246 (1982).

77. Sherwin R. Sudden death in men with increased risk of myocardial infarction. The MRFIT Programme. *Drugs 28* (Suppl. 1): 46–53 (1984).

78. Carone FA, Spector WG. The suppression of experimental proteinuria in the rat by compounds that inhibit increased capillary permeability. *J. Pathol. Bacteriol. 80*: 55–62 (1960).

79. Blantz RC, Konnen K. The mechanism of acute renal failure after uranyl nitrate. *J. Clin. Invest. 55*: 621–635 (1975).

80. Van Peer AP, Belpaire FM. Hepatic oxidative drug metabolism in rats with experimental renal failure. *Arch. Int. Pharmacodyn. Ther. 228*: 180–183 (1977).

81. Giacomini KM, Nakeeb SM, Levy G. Pharmacokinetic studies of propoxyphene I: effect of portacaval shunt on systemic availability in dogs. *J. Pharm. Sci. 69*: 786–789 (1980).

82. Waynforth HB. Animal operative techniques (in the mouse, rat, guinea pig and rabbit). In: Campbell PN, Sargent JR, eds. *Techniques in Protein Biosynthesis.* NY: Academic Press, Inc.; 1969: 209–249.

83. Klaassen CD. Comparison of the effects of two-thirds hepatectomy and bile duct ligation on hepatic excretory function. *J. Pharmacol. Exp. Ther. 191*: 25–31 (1974).

84. Meehan FP. Total hepatectomy in the rat. *Amer. J. Physiol. 179*: 282–284 (1954).

85. Mann FD, Shonyo ES, Mann FC. Effect of removal of the liver on blood coagulation. *Amer. J. Physiol. 164*: 111–116 (1951).

86. Pang KS, Gillette JR. A theoretical examination of the effects of gut wall metabolism, hepatic elimination, and enterohepatic recycling on estimates of bioavailability and of hepatic blood flow. *J. Pharmacokinet. Biopharm. 6*: 355–367 (1978).

87. Lee S, Chandler JG, Broelsch CE, Flamant YM, Orloff MJ. Portal-systemic anastomosis in the rat. *J. Surg. Res. 17*: 53–73 (1974).

88. Bircher J. The rat with portacaval shunt: an animal model with chronic hepatic failure. *Pharmacol. Ther. 5*: 219–222 (1979).

89. Agoston S, Houwertjes MC, Salt PJ. A new method for studying the relationship between hepatic uptake of drugs and their pharmacodynamic effects in anaesthetized cats. *Br. J. Pharmacol. 68*: 637–643 (1980).

90. Gugler R, Lain P, Azarnoff DL. Effect of portacaval shunt on the disposition of drugs with and without first-pass effect. *J. Pharmacol. Exp. Ther. 195*: 416–423 (1975).

91. Recknagel RO. Carbon tetrachloride hepatotoxicity. *Pharmacol. Rev. 19*: 145–208 (1967).

92. Klaassen CD, Plaa GL. Comparison of the biochemical alterations elicited in livers from rats treated with carbon tetrachloride, chloroform, 1,1,2-trichloroethane and 1,1,1-trichloroethane. *Biochem. Pharmacol. 18*: 2019–2027 (1969).

93. Koivusaari U, Lang M, Hietanen E. Differences in the response of hepatic and intestinal drug metabolizing enzymes in rats following carbon tetrachloride and/or phenobarbital treatment. *Acta Pharmacol. Toxicol. 46*: 37–42 (1980).

94. El-Hawari AM, Plaa GL. Impairment of hepatic mixed-function oxidase activity by alpha- and beta-naphthylisothiocyanate: relationship to hepatotoxicity. *Tox. Appl. Pharmacol. 48*: 445–458 (1979).

95. Downing RW, Rickels K, Meyers F. Side reactions in neurotics. I. A comparison of two methods of assessment. *J. Clin. Pharmacol. 10*: 289–297 (1970).

96. Howie JG, Clark GA. Double blind trial of early demethylchlortetracycline in minor respiratory illness in general practice. *Lancet 2*: 1099–1102 (1970).

97. Bulpitt CJ, Dollery CT, Carne S. A symptom questionaire of hypertensive patients. *J. Chronic Disease 27*: 309–323 (1974).

98. Avery CW, Ibelle BP, Allison B, Mandell N. Systematic errors in evaluation of side effects. *Amer. J. Psychiatry 123*: 875–878 (1967).

99. Aitken RCB. Measurement of feelings using visual analogue scales. *Proc. Roy. Soc. Med. 62*: 989–993 (1969).

100. Huskisson EC, Wojtulewski JA. Measurement of side effects of drugs. *Brit. Med. J. 2*: 698–699 (1974).

101. Lapierre YD. Evaluation des effets secondaires chez les neurotiques. Un essai avec les mesoridazins et le placebo. *Can. Psychiat. Assoc. J. 26*: 61–66 (1975).

102. New Zealand Hypertension Study Group. A multicentre open trial of labetalol in New Zealand. *Brit. J. Clin. Pharmacol. 8* (Suppl. 2): 179S–182S (1979).

103. Lasagna L. Bias in the elucidation of subjective side-effects. *Brit. J. Clin. Pharmacol. 11*: 111S–113 (1981).

104. Pearson RG, Byars GE. The development and validation of a checklist for measuring subjective fatigue. School of Aviation Medicine, USAF Report No. 56-115 (1956).

105. Glaser EM. Volunteers, controls, placebos and questionaires in clinical trials. In: Witts LJ, ed. *Medical Surveys and Clinical Trials*. London: Oxford University Press, Second Edition; 1964: 115–129.

106. Zealley AK, Aitken CB. Measurement of mood. *Proc. Roy. Soc. Med. 62*: 993–996 (1969).

107. Vinar O. Scale for rating treatment emergent symptoms in psychiatry DVP. *Activitas Nervosa Superior 13*: 238–240 (1971).

108. Anderson K, Malm U, Perris C, Rapp W, Roman G. The inter-rater reliability of scales for rating symptoms and side effects in schizophrenia patients during a clinical trial. *Acta Psychiat. Scand. 249* (Suppl.): 38–42 (1974).

109. Bond A, Lader M. The use of analogue scales in rating subjective feelings. *Brit. J. Med. Psychol. 47*: 211–218 (1974).

110. George CF. The investigation of new drugs in man. *Brit. J. Hosp. Med. 12*: 780–789 (1974).

111. Gagnon MA, Tebreault L. Pharmacologie humaine des anorexigenes. Validite d'un questionnaire sur l'appetit. *Un Med. Can. 104*: 922–929 (1975).

112. Huskisson EC. Assessment for clinical trials. *Clin. Rheumat. Dis. 2*: 37–49 (1976).

113. Laferriere N, Tenaillon A, Saltiel JC, Smagghe A, Chicon FJ, Chretien J, Portos JL. *Le questionnaire medical 1978.* Paris: Institut National de la Sante et de la Recherche Medicale, 1977.

114. U.S. Department of Health, Education and Welfare. Dosage record and treatment emergent symptom scale. In: *ECDEU Assessment Manual.* Washington, D.C.: U.S. Government Printing Office; 1976: 223–245.

115. McGavin CR, Artvinli M, Nave M, McHardy GJR. Dyspnoea, disability and distance walked. Comparison of estimates of exercise performance in respiratory disease. *Brit. Med. J. 2*: 241–243 (1978).

116. Lundberg PK. Assessments of drugs side effects. Visual analogue scale versus checklist format. *Perceptual and Motor Skills 50*: 1067–1073 (1980).

117. Levine J, Schooler N, Moynihan C. SAFTEE. A new method for assessing side effects in clinical trials. *Cont. Clin. Trials 4*: 157 (1983).

118. Greenblatt M. Controls in clinical research. *Clin. Pharmacol. Ther. 6*: 864–869 (1964).

119. Ciccolunghi SN, Chaudri HA. A methodological study of some factors influencing the reporting of symptoms. *J. Clin. Pharmacol. 15*: 496–505 (1975).

120. Cato AE, Cook L, Starbuck R, Heatherington D. Methodologic approach to adverse events applied to bupropion clinical trials. *J. Clin. Psychiatry 44*: 187–190 (1983).

121. Stephens MDB. *The Detection of New Adverse Drug Reactions.* New York: Stockton Press; 1985.

122. Bulpitt CJ. The evaluation of subjective well-being. In: *Randomized Controlled Clinical Trials.* The Hague: Martinus Nijhoff Publishers; 1983: 194–208.

123. Deyo RA. Measuring functional outcomes in therapeutic trials for chronic disease. *Controlled Clinical Trials 5*: 223–240 (1984).

124. Miller L, Dalton M, Vestal R, Perkins JG, Lyon G. Quality of life. I. Methodological and regulatory/scientific aspects. *J. Clin. Res. Drug Development 3*: 117–128 (1988).

125. Bulpitt CJ. Quality of life in hypertensive patients. In: Amery A, Fagard R, Lijnen P, Staessen J, eds. *Hypertensive Cardiovascular Disease: Patho-*

physiology and Treatment. The Hague: Martinus Nijhoff Publishers; Chapter 58, 1982: 929–948.

126. Jachuk SJ, Brierley H, Jachuk S, Willcox PM. The effect of hypotensive drugs on the quality of life. *J. Roy. Coll. Gen. Pract. 32*: 103–105 (1982).
127. McPeek B, Gilbert JP, Mosteller F. The end result: quality of life. In: Bunker JP, Barnes BA, Mosteller F, eds. *Costs, Risks, and Benefits of Surgery*. New York: Oxford University Press; 1977.
128. Fineberg HV, Hiatt HH. Evaluation of medical practices: the case for technology assessment. *N. Engl. J. Med. 301*: 1086–1091 (1979).
129. Mosteller F. Innovation and evaluation. *Science 211*: 811–816 (1981).
130. Coronary Artery Surgery Study (CASS). A randomized trial of coronary artery bypass surgery. Quality of life in patients randomly assigned to treatment groups. *Circulation 68*: 951–960 (1983).
131. Fayers PM, Jones DR. Measuring and analyzing quality of life in cancer clinical trials: a review. *Statistics in Medicine 2*: 429–446 (1983).
132. Wortman PM, Yeaton WH. Cumulating quality of life results in controlled trials of coronary artery bypass graft surgery. *Controlled Clinical Trials 6*: 289–305 (1985).
133. Karnovsky DA, Burchenal JH. The clinical evaluation of chemotherapeutic agents. In: Macleod CM, ed. *Symposium of New York Academy of Medicine, 1948*. New York: Columbia University Press; 1949.
134. Hyde L, Wolf J, McCracken S, Yesner R. Natural course of inoperable lung cancer. *Chest 64*: 309–312 (1973).
135. Dzau VJ, Colucci WS, Williams GH, Curfman G, Meggs L, Hollenberg NK. Sustained effectiveness of converting-enzyme inhibition in patients with severe congestive heart failure. *N. Engl. J. Med. 302*: 1373–1379 (1980).
136. Cohn LH, Mudge GH, Pratter F, Collins JJ. Five to eight-year follow-up of patients undergoing porcine heart valve replacement. *N. Engl. J. Med. 304*: 258–262 (1981).
137. Steinbrocker O, Traeger CH, Batterman RC. Therapeutic criteria in rheumatoid arthritis. *JAMA 140*: 659–662 (1979).
138. Cocchetto DM, Nardi RV. Benefit-risk assessment of investigational drugs: current methodology, limitations, and alternative approaches. *Pharmacotherapy 6*: 286–303 (1986).
139. Federal Food, Drug, and Cosmetic Act, As Amended. January, 1979. Section 505.

3

Limitations of Conventional Methods and Alternative Approaches to Benefit/Risk Assessment

> The origin of an original work is always
> the pursuit of a fact which does not
> fit into accepted ideas.
>
> *Claude Bernard*

I. LIMITATIONS OF CONVENTIONAL METHODS

Conventional approaches to benefit/risk assessment were described in the previous chapter. These conventional approaches are sub-optimal due to (1) conduct of safety assessments predominantly in clinical studies designed to assess efficacy, (2) insufficient attention to identification of the subpopulations of patients at uniquely high risk from the drug, and (3) experience with the drug in a study patient population which is much less heterogeneous than the general patient population that will receive the drug post-approval. The suboptimal nature of these methods of benefit/risk assessment is evident primarily in the periodic marketing of a drug with unacceptably high drug-associated risk. Unfortunately, the methodological limitations listed above can allow this unacceptable drug-associated risk to go undetected until after marketing. Indeed, there are a large number of drugs for which important drug-related toxicities were not detected until after marketing (Table 1).

On a related matter, the reader may have noted the implicit inference that the suboptimal nature of conventional methods of benefit/risk assessment is rarely manifested by periodic marketing of a drug with unacceptably low benefit. Such drugs rarely progress to marketing and, in fact,

Table 1. Tabulation of selected serious or catastrophic toxicities associated with drugs.

Toxicity	Associated Drug	Drug Class
Nephrotoxicities:		
Uric acid		
nephropathy	piroxicam [1]	NSAID
Acute Renal Failure	gentamicin [2–3]	antibacterial
	cephalexin [4]	antibacterial
	tetracycline [5]	antibacterial
	iodinated contrast media [6–8]	contrast dye
	amphotericin-B [9]	antifungal
Insterstitial	rifampicin [10–12]	antituberculin
Nephritis	methicillin [13]	antibacterial
Nephrogenic	lithium [14]	treatment of mania
Diabetes	chlorpropamide [15]	oral hypoglycemic agent
Insipidus	methoxyflurane [16]	anesthetic
Nephrotic	tolbutamide [17]	oral hypoglycemic agent
Syndrome	gold [18]	antirheumatic agent
	probenecid [19]	uricosuric
Hepatotoxicities:		
Acute hepatic injury	cimetidine [20]	H2-antagonist
	benoxaprofen [21–22]	NSAID
	zomepirac [23]	analgesic
	ticrynafen [24–25]	diuretic
Cholestatic injury	ranitidine [26]	H2-antagonist
Hemolytic Anemia	nomifensine [27]	antidepressant
Aplastic Anemia	chloramphenicol [28]	antibacterial
	phenylbutazone [29]	anti-inflammatory
	midazolam [30]	sedative/hypnotic
Seizure Disorders	penicillin G [31]	antibacterial
	maprotiline [32]	antidepressant
	lidocaine [31]	anesthetic, antiarrhythmic
	amitriptyline [33]	antidepressant
	bupropion	antidepressant
Ototoxicity	gentamicin [31]	antibacterial
Extrapyramidal	trifluoperazine [31]	antipsychotic
symptoms		
Phocomelia	thalidomide [34]	sedative/hypnotic
Oculomucocutaneous	practolol [35]	antihypertensive
syndrome		
Vaginal	diethyl stilboestrol [36]	synthetic estrogen
adenocarcinoma		

usually never result in a New Drug Application because the FDA, sponsors, statisticians, and investigators have invested a great deal of effort since the 1960s to develop vigorous standards for evidence of adequate benefit. Only later did the same vigor begin to be focused on standards for evidence of safety.

II. TWO ISSUES IN SAFETY ASSESSMENT

The safety profile of a drug must address two issues. The first issue is "catastrophic toxicity detection." This is indeed the supreme issue in terms of the ultimate adverse consequences of the drug to the public. The second issue in the safety profile is "selection of the dosage range."

Catastrophic toxicity includes potential lethality and other dramatic toxic manifestations such as hepatic necrosis, seizures, sudden cardiac death, agranulocytosis, and carcinogenicity. Prediction of these catastrophic toxicities is one principal goal of the extensive preclinical dose-response pharmacologic and toxicologic studies in a variety of animal species [37–44]. Administration of the drug to man in Phase I clinical trials may also detect catastrophic toxicities in the course of establishing the tolerable dose range in man. In both the preclinical toxicology research and the human Phase I dose-tolerance studies, a broad dose range is employed over a relatively broad duration of exposure (e.g., one dose to lifetime dosing in animals; one dose to up to 6 weeks in man) in order to facilitate detection of the acute and latent drug-induced illness or toxicity. Relatively small test populations can be employed because, at some dose, adverse events occur at a sufficiently high frequency compared to the frequency of such events in a placebo-control or untreated historical population [45]. Thus, the combination of frequent adverse events at some dose and easily identified clinical manifestations of toxicity render the detection of catastrophic toxicity inescapable. However, low frequency catastrophic events that are not dose-related are unlikely to be observed in these early studies. This is a limitation.

"Selection of the dose range," i.e., the second issue for consideration in the safety profile, consists of establishing dosage limits which provide an acceptable benefit/risk ratio [46]. Risk is assessed as clinical toxicities, including adverse events and functional abnormalities of major organs, as measured by clinical laboratory tests and physical examinations. This portion of the safety profile is performed in man. The conventional approach involves administering therapeutic doses of an investigational compound to a relatively large number of patients with the target disease and few, if any, concurrent complications (e.g., hepatic disease, hypothyroidism) during Phase II and III clinical trials. Patients are monitored before, during, and after therapy. Since patients have a relatively low incidence of major organ system dysfunction and pre-existing subjective complaints, the detection of treatment-emergent, potentially drug-associated adverse events (i.e., "signal") is facilitated by this setting of "low noise."

III. REASONS FOR INADEQUACIES OF SAFETY PROFILES

The sensitivity of the conventional benefit/risk approach seems suspect based on the reviewed data (Table 1). It appears that reasonable estimates of the true incidences and severities of the many renal, hepatic, neurologic, and hematologic toxicities associated with various therapies were not available until after marketing of many drugs. There appear to be two general reasons for this alarming incidence of suddenly discovered catastrophic toxicities. First, the diversity among patients receiving a given drug after it was marketed far exceeded the diversity among the patients receiving the drug during the investigational phases. Thus, the conventional safety assessment approach has limited value for defining the safe use of an efficacious compound among all of the subgroups of patients who are likely to receive it. Second, the conventional approach to safety assessment is to collect safety data as a *secondary* objective in efficacy studies. Considerable time and energy are routinely expended in efforts to design the efficacy components of prospective clinical trials. Methods of efficacy measurement are described in great detail in clinical protocols, as are the methods to be used in subsequent analyses of efficacy data. It is common to consider both the desired significance level and the desired power in calculating sample size for efficacy measures in clinical trials [47]. This same degree of prospective attention and planning is not commonly afforded to safety measures in clinical trials.

As a consequence, the major limitation of conventional safety assessment is that it can only detect safety concerns or toxicities occurring with considerable frequency in the subpopulations of patients who have diseases which are relatively uncomplicated. Of course, drug-induced illnesses in the patients enrolled in investigational drug studies may have frequencies close to the background frequencies of similar illnesses in an untreated or control population. The frequencies of many catastrophic toxicities are less than 0.1%. Quantitative similarity between the frequencies of potentially drug-associated events and background frequencies is observed for two reasons. First, subtle drug-related effects on previously healthy major organ systems may not produce an immediate, measurable change in either objective or subjective safety parameters (e.g., a decline in renal function as indicated by an increase in serum creatinine concentration). Second, few of the patients enrolled in investigational trials may be at increased risk of drug toxicity. For different drugs, different subpopulations of patients (e.g., patients with cirrhosis, elderly patients, or neonates) may be at dramatically increased risk. While such at-risk patients may experience a detectable change in some safety parameters in conventional clinical trials, the incidence of such changes will be diluted in the total clinical trial population, thereby remaining undetectably close to the background incidence. This deficiency can contribute to "suddenly discovered drug toxicities" during the period of post-marketing surveillance.

IV. ALTERNATIVE APPROACHES

There are specific methods that can be used to overcome these limitations. Alternative approaches are (1) complete exploration of an Integrated Summary of Safety, (2) more extensive safety testing of investigational drugs in patient populations at higher risk, and (3) assessment of safety in studies specifically designed to optimize safety evaluation. Such approaches serve the interest of patients, physicians, and drug developers by facilitating the development of new therapies through a more complete benefit/risk assessment prior to initial marketing of a new drug.

A. Integrated Summary of Safety

The first method is the event-oriented approach embodied in the Integrated Summary of Safety (ISS). The ISS became a required section of each New Drug Application with the NDA rewrites of 1985 [21 CFR 314.50 (d)(5)(vi)(a)]. The ISS uses the safety data collected via conventional benefit/risk methods, but it tries to minimize the limitations by asking sponsors and FDA medical officers to focus on those events most likely to be the "signal" for catastrophic toxicities. Those "signal events" are any patient who died during a clinical study and any patient who did not complete a clinical study because of an adverse event. Clearly, these two groups of patients met with two of the most severe outcomes of participation in a clinical trial. Careful and thorough examination of their data, on a patient-by-patient basis, has proven useful in detecting certain adverse events, thereby overcoming some of the limitations of conventional benefit/risk assessment. Dr. Temple [48] has provided a valuable summary of the historical evolution of the ISS. Drug developers are encouraged to use this tool to its full potential and to consider applying it in combination with other approaches.

B. Studies in Patient Subpopulations at Higher Risk

Historically, steps taken after an occurrence of a "suddenly discovered toxicity" with some drugs have identified a sub-population of patients for whom the risks of therapy are increased [45]. The safety-related limitations of the drug were then redefined [45]. In some cases, the drug was withdrawn from the market. In other cases, it was possible to exploit the efficacy of the compound in those patient subgroups with a desirably high benefit/ risk ratio. Since retrospective review has revealed evidence of some "suddenly discovered drug toxicities," it seems feasible to detect some of these toxicities and, in some cases, estimate their incidences from prospective studies. Such studies should be undertaken, in part, prior to marketing.

Discovery of a rare event can require study of a large population in order to have reasonable certainty of observation of the event in the presence of various background incidences (Table 2). However, benefit/risk assessment within a specific high-risk population greatly decreases the number of patients needed for observation (Table 2). While selection of the patient subgroups at risk may not always be done *a priori*, a reasonable place to begin is with the patient subgroups generally known to be at increased risk for a given disease, patient subgroups at increased risk of drug toxicity (e.g., pediatric or elderly patients), and patient subgroups having impaired function of the major organs of drug elimination. These major organs consist of the liver as the major organ for drug metabolism and the kidneys as the major organs for excretion of many drugs. Many abnormalities of drug disposition and elimination are well documented in these patient subgroups and drug-related adverse events for some drugs may be more likely in these patients with compromised major organ function. Therefore, benefit/risk of investigational drugs must be evaluated in patients with pre-existing major organ disease because of the possibilities of altered dose-response or dose-toxicity relationships.

For those subpopulations selected due to their potentially higher risk, the studies are relatively straightforward. An adequate number of patients from each particular subpopulation (e.g., major organ dysfunctions, concurrent diseases, or age) should be exposed to therapy with the investigational compound. Full safety and efficacy evaluations must be conducted.

Table 2. Number of patients necessary for study in order to detect adverse events with various incidences [49].

Background Incidence of Adverse Event	Additional Incidence of Adverse Event on Drug		
	1 in 100	1 in 1,000	1 in 10,000
1 in 10	20,000	2,000,000	200,000,000
1 in 100	3,200	220,000	22,000,000
1 in 1000	1,300	32,000	2,300,000

Patients with relatively stable disease provide a stable baseline on which to detect manifestations of drug-induced illnesses. Such patients may also require concurrent medications which may alter the safety and efficacy of the investigational drug. The possibility of such interactions can be studied. These evaluations will enable formulation of an adequate benefit/risk assessment and provide the information required to intelligently use the new drug.

Importantly, the design and analysis of clinical studies in such selected subpopulations are straightforward. Further, these studies can be conducted with a reasonably homogeneous group of patients. Such homogeneity is not achievable in the enormous, multinational Phase IV studies that some investigators and sponsors implement with the hope of discovering serious, low frequency adverse events. Studying small numbers of patients from selected subpopulations seems the preferable approach when drug-associated risk can reasonably be predicted in relationship to a specific patient characteristic (e.g., patient age). However, use of a large heterogeneous population in a Phase IV post-marketing surveillance study may be a preferred approach to characterize effects in a broad population when no particular subpopulation is suspected of being at uniquely high risk.

Recently, there has been increasing attention to the possibility of increased risk of drug toxicity in selected subpopulations of patients. Population pharmacokinetic studies have been proposed as a means to discern a need for dosage regimen alterations for various patient subpopulations [50]. With this approach, the plasma drug concentration versus time profiles of a population of patients with reduced renal or hepatic function, for example, are compared with similar profiles from a population of patients with normal organ function. Based on these comparative clinical pharmacokinetic properties, dosage regimens are altered for patients with renal or hepatic impairment to produce the same therapeutic effect as the subjects with normal organ function. This approach can reduce the risks for patients with major organ dysfunction. However, the studies must have a sufficient duration of treatment to assess subjective and objective safety parameters. Such studies in patients with major organ dysfunction must also assess drug toxicities in organs other than the one that is impaired. For example, patients with reduced renal function may have significant changes in the pharmacokinetic properties of a drug which is metabolized outside of the kidneys or bound to non-renal proteins [51–53]. An increased proportion of unbound drug may markedly increase toxicity of the compound and at the same time produce changes in other pharmacokinetic parameters. Finally, population studies must characterize the concurrent pharmacodynamic properties of the drug since the pharmacodynamic properties determine the benefits of therapy. Such concurrent pharmacokinetic and pharmacodynamic characterizations can facilitate clinical drug development. This approach has been advocated by some at FDA and it has already played a role in FDA's review of one drug, ketoralac [54].

C. Studies Designed Specifically to Assess Safety

Throughout the 1960s and 1970s, FDA, investigators, and sponsors were keenly focused on testing and refining ways to characterize efficacy of various drugs. This focus followed the Kefauver-Harris Amendments in 1962 which mandated substantial evidence of efficacy prior to approval of a new drug. There are few instances where comparable effort has been focused on developing study designs specifically to characterize the safety profiles of drugs. Clearly, studies can be designed specifically to detect a certain frequency of an uncommon adverse event or detect a difference in frequency of an adverse event from control. Studies can also be designed to characterize the time course of emergence of adverse events after withdrawal of a drug or the time course of resolution of events after discontinuation of a drug. Studies can be designed to look specifically at the safety profile of combination regimens. Clearly, the safety profile of zidovudine-based combination regimens will be a major determinant of whether such combination regimens can be used in certain patients with AIDS.

In some cases, studies that are specific to safety issues may yield results that enable a drug to be marketed. For example, it is not clear that Burroughs Wellcome Co. would have ever been able to market bupropion (Wellbutrin®) without a safety study. As described in the product's package insert, 25 of approximately 2400 bupropion-treated patients in the original NDA program experienced seizures [55]. The frequency of seizures appeared to increase substantially with increasing dose. Subsequently, a separate prospective study was designed to focus specifically at the incidence of seizures among patients treated for 8 weeks at doses up to the maximum recommended daily dose (450 mg per day). This study showed 8 seizures in 8 weeks of treatment among approximately 3200 patients. The finding that the frequency of seizures was limited to $< 0.4\%$ with doses ≤ 450 mg/day was a critical finding that enabled marketing of the drug with appropriate directions for its use.

A second example illustrates how knowledge of a new drug's risks can have a dramatic effect on its safe use. Clozapine (Clozaril®, Sandoz) is an atypical antipsychotic agent that can provide great benefit to certain schizophrenic patients. Unfortunately, clozapine has been associated with severe granulocytopenia and agranulocytosis. According to the product's package insert, knowledge of clozapine-induced agranulocytosis became more widespread in 1977 [56]. Before that time, 112 cases of agranulocytosis were reported worldwide in association with clozapine and 35% of these cases were fatal. After 1977, few cases were fatal because patients underwent close monitoring of leukocytes. The cumulative incidence at 1 year of agranulocytosis (polys + bands less than 500 per mm^3) has been estimated as approximately 1.3%. In view of this frequency and the potential for fatality if not detected early, Sandoz initially supplied clozapine only through the Clozaril Patient Management System (CPMS). CPMS is a system for dispensing the drug only to patients who agree to have weekly leukocyte counts. Any patient who refuses this frequent monitoring to facilitate early detection of granulocytopenia will not receive clozapine. Clearly, the cost to the patient of CPMS is substantial at an estimated $172 per week [57]. However, clozapine would probably not be approved in the U.S. without a means of protecting patients from the substantial risk of agranulocytosis. The protection provided by CPMS enables the drug-related antipsychotic benefits to be provided to patients who are willing to receive the drug in the lower-risk environment provided by CPMS.

D. Summary of Alternative Approaches

We have described three alternative methods of benefit/risk assessment for new drugs. Of course, these three methods are not mutually exclusive. There is overlap, for example, between designing a study to assess a safety issue and electing to focus that study on a patient subpopulation at higher risk. Also, the event-oriented approach to analysis of safety data in the Integrated Summary of Safety is a valuable approach to use in reviewing any collection of safety data. We advocate combination of multiple approaches to collect and analyze safety data because, for many drugs, you cannot be sure what event you are looking for until you find it. This necessity to use multiple approaches is less pressing with efficacy data since the desirable outcome is a significant finding. Clearly, demonstrating the *occurrence* of a frequent, significant efficacy finding is a very different exercise than demonstrating the *absence* of an infrequent, significant safety finding. Since the desirable outcome of safety assessment is no significant finding, drug developers increase their confidence in this non-finding by using multiple approaches concurrently.

REFERENCES

1. Pulliam JP, Mundis RJ, Muther RS. Piroxicam (Feldene) predisposes to chemotherapy-induced acute uric acid nephropathy. *Arthritis and Rheumatism 27*: 116–117 (1984).
2. Kahn T, Stein RM. Gentamicin and renal failure. *Lancet 1*: 498 (1972).

3. Gary NE, Buzzeo L, Salaki J, Eisinger RP. Gentamicin-associated acute renal failure. *Arch. Intern. Med. 136*: 1101–1104 (1976).
4. Fung-Herrera CG, Mulvaney WP. Cephalexin nephrotoxicity. Reversible nonoliguric acute renal failure and hepatotoxicity associated with cephalexin therapy. *JAMA 229*: 318–319 (1974).
5. Phillips ME, Eastwood JB, Curtis JR, Gower PE, DeWardener HE. Tetracycline poisoning in renal failure. *Br. Med. J. 2*: 149–151 (1974).
6. Bergman LA, Ellison MR, Dunea G. Acute renal failure after drip-infusion pyelography. *N. Engl. J. Med. 279*: 1277 (1968).
7. Hanaway J, Black J. Renal failure following contrast injection for computerized tomography. *JAMA 238*: 2056 (1977).
8. Wagoner RD. Acute renal failure associated with contrast agents. *Arch. Intern. Med. 138*: 353 (1978).
9. Bennett JE, Brandriss MW, Butler WT, Hill GJ. Amphotericin B toxicity. Combined clinical staff conference at the National Institutes of Health. *Ann. Intern. Med. 61*: 334–354 (1964).
10. Poole G, Stradling P, Worlledge S. Potentially serious side effects of high-dose twice-weekly rifampicin. *Br. Med. J. 3*: 343–347 (1971).
11. Campese VM, Marzullo F, Schena FP, Coratelli P. Acute renal failure during intermittent rifampicin therapy. *Nephron 10*: 256–261 (1973).
12. Rothwell DL, Richmond DE. Hepatorenal failure with self-initiated intermittent rifampicin therapy. *Br. Med. J. 2*: 481–482 (1974).
13. Galpin JE, Shinaberger JH, Stanley TM, Blumenkrantz MJ, Bayer AS, Friedman GS, Montgomerie JZ, Guze LB, Coburn JW, Glassock RJ. Acute interstitial nephritis due to methicillin. *Amer. J. Med. 65*: 756–765 (1978).
14. Lee RV, Jampol LM, Brown WV. Nephrogenic diabetes insipidus and lithium intoxication—complications of lithium carbonate therapy. *N. Engl. J. Med. 284*: 93–94 (1971).
15. Garcia M, Miller M, Moses AM. Chlorpropamide-induced water retention in patients with diabetes mellitus. *Ann. Int. Med. 75*: 549–554 (1971).
16. Mazze RI, Shue GL, Jackson SH. Renal dysfunction associated with methoxyflurane anesthesia. A randomized prospective clinical evaluation. *JAMA 216*: 278–288 (1971).
17. Schnall C, Wiener JS. Nephritis occurring during tolbutamide administration. *JAMA 167*: 214–215 (1958).
18. Silverberg DS, Kidd EG, Shnitka TK, Ulan RA. Gold nephropathy. A clinical and pathologic study. *Arthritis Rheum. 13*: 812–825 (1970).
19. Sokol A, Bashner MH, Okun R. Nephrotic syndrome caused by probenecid. *JAMA 199*: 43–44 (1967).
20. Van Steenbergen W, Vanstapel MJ, Desmet V, Vankerckvoorde L, DeKeyzer R, Brijs R, Fevery J, DeGroote J. Cimetidine-induced liver injury. Report of three cases. *J. Hepatology 1*: 359–368 (1985).
21. Goudie BM, Birnie GF, Watkinson G, MacSween RNM, Kissen LH, Cunningham NE. Jaundice associated with the use of benoxaprofen. *Lancet 1*: 959 (1982).

22. Hamdy RC, Murname B, Perera N, Woodcock K, Koch IM. The pharmacokinetics of benoxaprofen in elderly subjects. *Eur. J. Rheumatol. Inflamm.* 5: 69–75 (1982).
23. Ruoff GE, Andelman SY, Cannella JJ. Long-term safety of zomepirac: a double-blind comparison with aspirin in patients with osteoarthritis. *J. Clin. Pharmacol.* 20: 377–384 (1980).
24. Lafay JP, Poupon R, Legendre C, Homberg JC, Darnis F. Hepatic lesions associated with antimicrosomal antibodies of the liver and kidney (type 2) and the taking of tienilic acid. A study of 37 cases. *Gastroenterol. Clin. Biol.* 7: 523–528 (1983).
25. Zimmerman HJ, Lewis JH, Ishak KG, Maddrey WC. Ticrynafen-associated hepatic injury: analysis of 340 cases. *Hepatology 4*: 315–323 (1984).
26. Colin-Jones DG. Comparison of ranitidine, 150 mg twice daily, with ranitidine, 300 mg in one evening dose, in the treatment of duodenal ulcer. In: *Ranitidine Therapeutic Advances* (Misiewicz JJ, Wood JR, eds.). Amsterdam: Excerpta Medica, 1984, Chapter 7, pp. 140–153.
27. Hoechst-Roussel merital (nomifensine) worldwide market withdrawal follow reported increase in incidence of severe hemolytic anemia adverse reactions. *FDC Reports 48*: 3 (1986).
28. Baumelou E, Najean Y. Why still prescribe chloramphenicol in 1983? Comparison of the clinical and biological hematologic effects of chloramphenicol and thiamphenicol. *Blut 47*: 317–320 (1983).
29. Heit WF. Hematologic effects of antipyretic analgesics. Drug-induced agranulocytosis. *Amer. J. Med. 75*: 65–69 (1983).
30. Anonymous. Death of a volunteer. *Br. Med. J. 290*: 1369–1370 (1985).
31. Porter J, Jick H. Drug-induced anaphylaxis, convulsions, deafness, and extrapyramidal symptoms. *Lancet 1*: 587–588 (1977).
32. Edwards JG, Glen-Bott M. Mianserin and convulsive seizures. *Br. J. Clin. Pharmacol. 15*: 299S–311S (1983).
33. Peck AW, Stern WC, Watkinson C. Incidence of seizures during treatment with tricyclic antidepressant drugs and bupropion. *J. Clin. Psychiatry 44*: 197–201 (1983).
34. Distillers Company (Biochemicals Ltd.). Distaval. *Lancet 2*: 1262 (1961).
35. Wright P. Untoward effects associated with practolol administration: oculomucocutaneous syndrome. *Br. Med. J. 1*: 595–598 (1975).
36. Herbst AL, Ulfelder H, Poskanzer DC. Adenocarcinoma of the vagina. Association of maternal stilboestrol therapy with tumour appearance in young women. *N. Engl. J. Med. 284*: 878–881 (1971).
37. Peck HM. An appraisal of drug safety evaluation in animals and the extrapolation of results to man. In: Tedeschi DH, Tedeschi RE, eds. *Importance of Fundamental Principles in Drug Evaluation*. New York: Raven Press, pp. 449–471 (1968).
38. Stevenson DE. Current problems in the choice of animals for toxicity testing. *J. Toxicol. Environ. Health 5*: 9–15 (1979).
39. Briggs GB, Oehme FW. Toxicology. In: Baker HJ, Lindsey JR, Weisbroth

SH, eds. *The Laboratory Rat. Volume II. Research Applications*. New York: Academic Press, pp. 103–118 (1980).

40. Bradner WT, Schurig JE. Toxicology screening in small animals. *Cancer Treatment Reviews 8*: 93–102 (1981).
41. Grahame-Smith DG. Preclinical toxicological testing and safeguards in clinical trials. *Europ. J. Clin. Pharmacol. 22*: 1–6 (1982).
42. CIOMS (The Council for International Organizations of Medical Sciences). *Safety Requirements for the First Use of New Drugs and Diagnostic Agents in Man. A Review of Safety Issues in Early Clinical Trials of Drugs*. Geneva: CIOMS, 1983.
43. Traina VM. The role of toxicology in drug research and development. *Medicinal Research Reviews 3*: 43–72 (1983).
44. Kapeghian JC, Traina VM. The role of experimental toxicology in safety evaluation: challenges facing the pharmaceutical industry. *Medicinal Research Reviews 10*: 271–280 (1990).
45. Jick H. The discovery of drug-induced illness. *N. Engl. J. Med. 296*: 481–485 (1977).
46. Finkel MJ. Important considerations for the clinical evaluation of drugs: appropriate dosing regimens. *Drug Intell. Clin. Pharm. 18*: 256–258 (1984).
47. Freiman JA, Chalmers TC, Smith H, Kuebler RR. The importance of beta, the type II error and sample size in the design and interpretation of the randomized control trial. *N. Engl. J. Med. 299*: 690–694 (1978).
48. Temple RJ. The regulatory evolution of the integrated safety summary. *Drug Information Journal* (in press).
49. Lewis JA. Post-marketing surveillance: how many patients? *Trends in Pharmacological Sciences 2*: 93–94 (1981).
50. Sheiner LB, Benet LZ. Premarketing observational studies of population pharmacokinetics of new drugs. *Clin. Pharmacol. Ther. 38*: 481–587 (1985).
51. Bennett WM, Aronoff GR, Morrison G, Golper TA, Pulliam J, Wolfson M, Singer I. Drug prescribing in renal failure: dosing guidelines for adults. *Amer. J. Kidney Dis. 3*: 155–193 (1983).
52. Brater DC, Chennavasin P. Effects of renal disease: pharmacokinetic considerations. In: Benet LZ, Massoud N, Gambertoglio JG, eds. *Pharmacokinetic Basis for Drug Treatment*. New York: Raven Press, pp. 119–147 (1984).
53. Gambertoglio JG. Effects of renal disease: altered pharmacokinetics. In: Benet LZ, Massoud N, Gambertoglio JG, eds. *Pharmacokinetic Basis for Drug Treatment*. New York: Raven Press, pp. 149–171 (1984).
54. Presentation by Dr. Carl C. Peck. *Dickinson's FDA 6* (Number 7): 1 (April 15, 1990).
55. Package insert for Wellbutrin®. *Physicians' Desk Reference*. Oradell, N.J.: Medical Economics Co. Inc., 45th Edition, 1991.
56. Package insert for Clozaril®. *Physicians' Desk Reference*. Oradell, N.J.: Medical Economics Co. Inc., 45th Edition, 1991.
57. Prager K. Clozaril: Torts' dangerous side effects. *The Wall Street Journal*, page A-18 (December 6, 1990).

4

Principles of Dose-Response Relationships with Application to Clinical Drug Development

> Poisons and medicine are oftentimes
> the same substance given with
> different intents.
>
> *Peter Mere Latham*

I. INTRODUCTION

A. The Phases of Clinical Drug Development

Historically, clinical drug development has been described as a sequential process. The pre-approval segments are known as Phases I–III, despite the obvious difficulty in defining clear separations between phases [1]. The recent IND rewrites refined the historical definitions of these phases and, while there is recognition that the phase separations are not distinct, some attempt was made to retain the three phases of premarketing clinical drug development. The IND rewrites defined the investigational phases as follows [2]:

(a) Phase 1

(1) Phase 1 includes the initial introduction of an investigational new drug into humans. Phase 1 studies are typically closely monitored and may be conducted in patients or normal volunteer subjects. These studies are designed to determine the metabolism and pharmacologic actions of the drug in humans, the side effects associated with increasing doses, and if possible, to gain early evidence on effectiveness. During Phase 1, sufficient information

about the drug's pharmacokinetics and pharmacologic effects should be obtained to permit the design of well-controlled, scientifically valid, Phase 2 studies. The total number of subjects and patients included in Phase 1 studies varies with the drug, but is generally in the range of 20 to 80.

(2) Phase 1 studies also include studies of drug metabolism, structure-activity relationships and mechanism of action in humans as well as studies in which investigational drugs are used as research tools to explore biological phenomena or disease processes.

(b) Phase 2

Phase 2 includes the controlled clinical studies conducted to evaluate the effectiveness of the drug for a particular indication or indications in patients with the disease or condition under study and to determine the common short-term side effects and risks associated with the drug. Phase 2 studies are typically well controlled, closely monitored, and conducted in a relatively small number of patients, usually involving no more than several hundred subjects.

(c) Phase 3

Phase 3 studies are expanded controlled and uncontrolled trials. They are performed after preliminary evidence suggesting effectiveness of the drug has been obtained and are intended to gather the additional information about effectiveness and safety that is needed to evaluate the overall benefit-risk relationship of the drug and to provide an adequate basis for physician labeling. Phase 3 studies usually include from several hundred to several thousand subjects.

B. The Dose-Response Perspective in Drug Development

The preceding definitions of the three phases of clinical drug development provide a broad view of the overall process. Obviously, drug development must proceed from tightly supervised, scientifically vigorous studies in relatively small groups of homogeneous subjects in Phase I to more realistic, systematic studies in much larger groups of far more heterogeneous patients in Phase III. Along this progressive path, knowledge of the relationship between dose of the drug and response of various patients must be accurately collected. To understand the intent of characterizing dose-response relationships, the fundamental question posed in any clinical drug study must be reviewed.

The drug development process consists of a continuous effort to improve the overall knowledge base on use of the new chemical entity (NCE) for treatment of human disease [3–5]. The intellectual basis for this continuum concept is that, throughout the drug development process, there is actually only one question being asked: *What does this compound do?* Moreover, the answer to this question is *always* formed as a dose-response evaluation, i.e., the NCE has "y units" activity at "x dose." As a practical matter, drug development consists of a series of questions in the form, "What does this compound do to _____ ?" where the blank specifies an organ system (e.g., kidneys) or research area (e.g., toxicology) that can contribute to the overall assessment of potential benefits and risks of a NCE. Obviously, at any point in this process when it becomes clear that the overall benefits provided by the drug do not outweigh the risks, the compound should be withdrawn from further development.

The majority of NCEs do not progress into clinical studies from prior preclinical evaluations. Such preclinical studies center on identification of the pharmacologic and toxicologic activity of the NCE. Initially, the discovery effort will focus on an evaluation of the so-called primary pharmacology of an NCE. The primary pharmacology consists of characterization of the effects of the drug on its target organ systems. For example, primary pharmacology of a potential antidepressant drug would usually include assessment of effects on principal animal models of depression and assessment of cardiovascular effects. Compounds with the desired primary pharmacological profile progress through the preclinical evaluation, including secondary pharmacology and toxicology [4,6], while compounds without the desired pharmacological profile never progress to clinical trials. To conduct these preclinical evaluations, the effect of a compound is ordinarily measured on major organ systems and on animal models of target diseases and non-target diseases; then, an attempt is made to identify the overall toxicity of the compound in the whole animal. A series of experiments is designed to identify the dose-response profile for a compound on a variety of parameters related to the activity of the organ system or disease of interest. For example, a cardiovascular assessment would include studies of blood pressure, heart rate, cardiac rhythm, and cardiac output. For a neuropharmacological evaluation, electrophysiologic activity and behavioral parameters may be studied. Each such assessment yields a dose-response profile (Figure 1). Comparison of these dose-response profiles enables a determination of whether the dose-response curve for the desirable pharmacological activity is to the left (i.e., at lower doses) of the dose-response curve for the undesirable toxic activity.

The experiment and types of answers are the same when testing drugs in man. Namely, we address "what the drug does" by experimentally

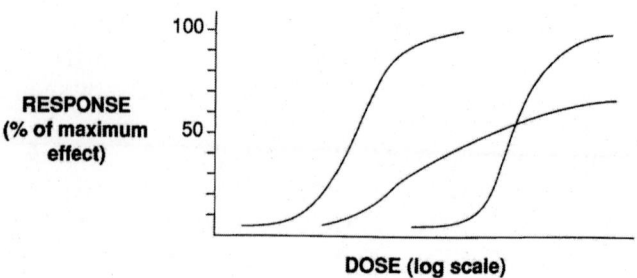

Figure 1. Comparison of multiple dose-response curves in animals for cardiovascular effect, gastrointestinal effect, and CNS effect.

characterizing a series of dose-response curves. Ultimately, the overall benefit/risk assessment is formed by comparing the steady-state dose-response curves for therapeutic benefits with the steady-state dose-response curves for undesirable, toxic effects (risks) (Figure 2). The relationship between the therapeutic dose-response curve and the toxic dose-response curve for a given NCE is studied over a range of doses called the *investigational dose range*. Then, as experience and understanding increase regarding the relationship between efficacy and toxicity dose-response curves, use of the NCE can expand into larger patient populations to allow definition of a *therapeutic dose range* and ultimately the optimal therapeutic regimen for a given patient population.

II. INVESTIGATIONAL DOSE RANGE

A. Definition and Importance

Embarking on large-scale clinical trials without a fundamental appreciation of the relationships between therapeutic and toxic dose-response

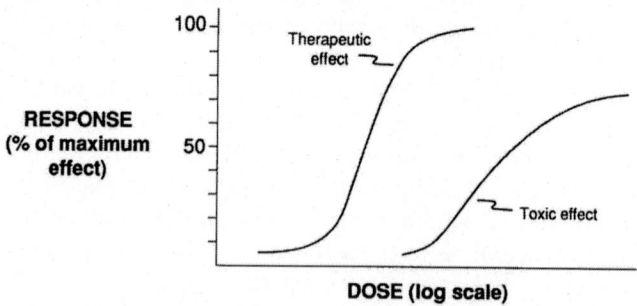

Figure 2. Comparison of dose-response curves for therapeutic effect (benefit) and toxic effect (risk).

curves is not rational. Consequently, the initial clinical trials on a NCE should be small with the objective of establishing the investigational dose range. A variety of study designs can be used for this purpose, depending on the specific drug class [7–10]. The *investigational dose range is defined as the breadth of doses bounded at the minimum by the "maximum no-effect dose" and bounded at the top by the "maximum tolerated dose"* (Figure 3). The maximum tolerated dose is a dose at which there is unequivocal evidence of an unacceptable frequency or severity of clinically significant adverse experiences. The subjects need not become frankly ill, but rather the observation of a consistent untoward change from baseline would be sufficient. Identification of the maximum tolerable dose is one of the primary purposes of initial clinical trials; as a result, these studies are often referred to as dose-tolerance studies. The purpose of early identification of maximum tolerated dose is to discern a dose above which patients need not be exposed in subsequent studies. Some may argue that these "dose-tolerance" studies also help identify the adverse events likely to be associated with the NCE in patients. It seems rather pedestrian to assert that making healthy volunteers sick in an escalating dose-tolerance study is a scientifically effective means to identify potential adverse events in patients. Further, a scientifically rigorous clinical pharmacology assessment across organ systems in the investigational dose range and preferably conducted in patients should provide far more useful information about potential drug-induced illnesses [11]. This is the analog in the clinical development phase of the dose-ranging studies in the preclinical phase. Without the latter, no one would accept that there was a reasonable basis for proceeding to the first human study. Similarly, appropriate dose-ranging studies in man provide a vital part of the reasonable basis for proceeding to expanded clinical studies.

The maximum no-effect dose is more problematic to characterize, although it is vital to subsequent development of the compound. Obviously,

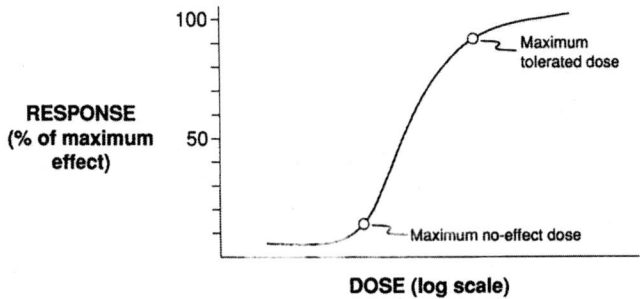

Figure 3. Investigational dose range.

it is possible to identify a dose with no activity, but we really need to know a dose which barely misses being active or has only a small fraction of the maximum achievable pharmacologic activity. The error made most often is to characterize an excessively high dose as the maximum no-effect dose or simply fail to study the matter. Since most investigators and sponsors dread the possibility of giving too little of a new drug, failure to rigorously identify this low end of the investigational dose range will skew subsequent clinical studies toward use of excessive doses and, thereby, increase the likelihood that the doses selected as optimal will be higher than necessary. In addition, such excessive doses may not be ultimately approvable.

Thus, identification of initial clinical trials with the nomenclature dose-tolerance trials may inappropriately focus on identification of the maximum tolerated dose, while obscuring the equally important determination of the maximum no-effect dose. Importantly, the notion that the investigational dose range can be identified in a single study of relatively few subjects (e.g., 20) receiving single doses of a NCE may be misguided. Initial clinical trials must focus on thoroughly characterizing the investigational dose range in order to provide the optimal chance of a subsequent decision-enabling clinical development program. To many, this point seems obvious, but it is emphasized in view of the large number of drug development programs that are built on a foundation of wholly inadequate dose-response information.

B. Some Practical Considerations

One possible practical approach to determining the investigational dose range is to identify in humans some analogues of the pharmacological activities that were sensitively detected in preclinical evaluations. Consequently, some attention must be paid to the potential to monitor the same parameters in both animals and man. This approach can be helpful for identification of both ends of the investigational dose range. While this approach will require considerable interaction between the preclinical and clinical project teams, it is important enough to merit such interaction, even though many compounds may never progress to the clinic.

Interaction between the preclinical and clinical project teams also may facilitate initial development of the clinical benefit/risk profile which begins with early clinical trials [5,11,12]. These early trials investigate a broad dose range in a limited group of subjects, many of whom may be healthy volunteers. These studies often require intense subject monitoring of many parameters deemed to be indicative of the activities and toxicities identified in preclinical evaluation of the compound. Obviously, the total experience (i.e., number of subjects) at any given dose will be small. Consequently, identification of the maximum tolerated dose will be affected by observations representing fairly large changes in physiology that occur with frequencies of at least 3-10%. These changes represent the obvious risks or limiting toxicities that must be anticipated in subsequent trials and minimized by selecting the appropriate therapeutic dose range. It is not certain that these events represent the adverse events that patients will experience in the later clinical trials.

The limited sensitivity of these early trials to small changes in patient-frequency of adverse events dictates a conservative approach in the conduct and interpretation of these trials. In this case, conservatism means we can more safely accept underestimates of both dose boundaries for the investigational dose range. As studies expand into patients with more complex pathology, avoiding pharmacotherapy-associated risk will be important and low pharmacotherapy-associated benefit may actually be sufficient for patients with milder disease in initial efficacy studies [11,13,14].

III. THERAPEUTIC DOSE RANGE

A. Definition and Importance

Once an investigational dose range is established, the next step is to identify that narrower portion of this range comprising the therapeutic dose range. This is the steady-state dose range over which the therapeutic efficacy of the compound is apparent while the adverse experiences are at an acceptably low level. *The therapeutic dose range is defined as the breadth of doses bounded at the minimum by the "minimum effective dose" and bounded at the top by the "maximum therapeutic dose"* (Figure 4). Determination of the therapeutic dose range requires elucidation of both the dose range where therapeutic effects are observed and the dose range where adverse experiences are observed. Ideally, the therapeutic dose range is the range where the desirable pharmacologic activity of the compound increases in a dose-dependent manner while the toxicity curve remains

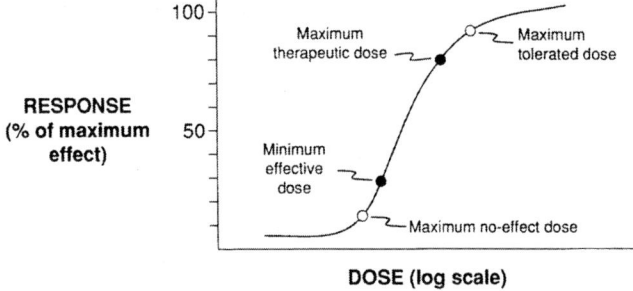

Figure 4. Comparison of therapeutic dose range with investigational dose range.

unchanged near zero. The top of the therapeutic dose range (i.e., "maximum therapeutic dose") is defined by the lower of either (1) the dose which shows clinically significant increases in untoward effects or (2) the dose above which further increases in therapeutic efficacy are not significant. It is important that the top "flat" portion of the classical sigmoidal efficacy dose-response curve is not commonly part of the therapeutic dose range. The slow asymptotic rise in this portion of the dose-response curve is usually indicative of subpopulation variability rather than a broader therapeutic dose range.

Hopefully, the therapeutic and toxic dose ranges will be separable; otherwise, the compound can not be developed unless it is targeted at life-threatening diseases for which there are currently no adequate therapies. Identifying doses that can produce therapeutic benefit should not be difficult since the compound was selected for development based on its possession of such activity. The difficulty lies in the precision of determination of the maximum therapeutic dose. In most cases, the maximum therapeutic dose should be less than the maximum tolerated dose. Thus, as clinical pharmacology studies progress in the target patient population, identification of a dose which produces none of the effects that contributed to determining the maximum tolerated dose should be the first approximation of the maximum therapeutic dose. If the efficacy and toxicity curves are not clearly separable, then the maximum therapeutic dose will be determined by identifying the dose at which unacceptable adverse experiences are observed, even if this dose does not provide maximum therapeutic activity (Figure 5). There may be subpopulations of patients where further increases in therapeutic activity may be important enough to warrant acceptance of increased toxicity, but that question should not be addressed until after the therapeutic dose range is well understood. Also, there may be sub-

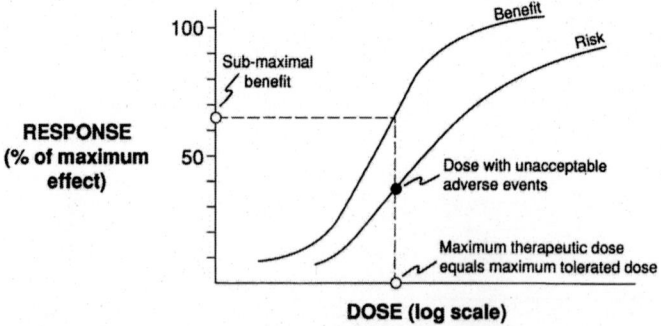

Figure 5. Example of a dose limited by the presence of unacceptable adverse events, despite achievement of sub-maximal benefit.

populations of patients with greater separation between efficacy and toxicity dose-response curves. Here, characterization of the therapeutic dose range will be easier. If the efficacy and toxicity dose-response curves are widely separated, the initial approximation of maximum therapeutic dose may be on the "flat" maximal response portion of the dose-response curve. This occurs with some antibacterial drugs. As indicated above, such a dose is usually outside the therapeutic dose range. Thus, the challenge is to determine the dose which achieves 80-90% of the maximum achievable therapeutic activity. Identifying this dose will facilitate determination of whether further increases in dose produce significant therapeutic gain. This, in turn, reinforces the experimental determination of maximum therapeutic dose.

B. Limiting the Maximum Therapeutic Dose

Some courage must be exercised to conclude that increasing doses do not significantly increase benefit. This courage is required for two reasons. First, it is difficult clinically to ignore even marginal increases in therapeutic benefit (e.g., doubling the dose provides a 5% increase in response). However, it is important to focus on identification of a realistic therapeutic dose range that can be used for subsequent clinical development in the large, more heterogeneous patient population that will enter Phase III studies. Later studies, perhaps in Phase IV, of patient subpopulations may identify particular utility of doses above the therapeutic dose range. Second, the higher doses increase the risk of side effects in subsequent studies in patients who are probably not as healthy and certainly more heterogenous than patients participating in the clinical pharmacology portion of the development program.

C. Characterization of Minimum Effective Dose

Accurate characterization of the low end of the dose-response curve represents the biggest practical problem in elucidating both the investigational dose range and therapeutic dose range. It is obviously difficult to detect pharmacologic activities that are only slightly above background. Theoretically, the pharmacologic activity of a NCE that confers benefit is observed at lower doses than the doses associated with adverse experiences. Thus, the low end of the investigational dose range (i.e., maximum no-effect dose) can help guide the initial approximation of minimum effective dose. Also, identification of doses that produce graded, but submaximal, alteration of the pharmacologic endpoints can aid characterization of minimum effective dose. Of course, a dose that produces 20-50% of the maximum achievable pharmacologic effect is not necessarily the minimum effective dose. Acceptance of this view will guard against skewing the therapeutic dose range toward higher doses.

Knowledge of the low end of the therapeutic dose range may permit controlled clinical studies in settings where a placebo control is not acceptable. A dose at the low end of the therapeutic dose range has some benefit and may enable a dose-ranging design that can facilitate regulatory approval. This low end of the dose-response curve may also be important when the efficacy and toxicity curves are not easily separable at other doses. If toxicity is present even at doses that provide minimal therapeutic benefit, then approval of the drug would be limited to very special circumstances. Clinical studies of a low dose in the hypothesized therapeutic dose range may provide the acid test of whether a NCE can be approvable in the patient population under study.

D. Conservative Selection of Therapeutic Dose Range

Implicit in identification of the therapeutic dose range is the notion that the benefits of therapy outweigh the risks for some portion of the target patient population when administered the drug within some dose range. Obviously, the cumulative experience will still be fairly limited at the end of Phase II when the therapeutic dose range is chosen. The limit of detection of occurrence of adverse experiences is in the 1–3% range for Phase II studies with 100–200 patients. With such high limits of detection, we must be conservative about identification of the minimum effective dose. Similarly, we must remain conservative in characterizing the maximum therapeutic dose since catastrophic toxicities (usually with less than 1% frequency) would represent major impediments to successful development of the NCE [11,13,14]. Since identifying the therapeutic dose range may be the most important portion of the clinical drug development program, it should be complete and rational. Expanded experience and improved confidence gained in this portion of the clinical program will have multiplicative impact on the quality of subsequent clinical trials.

IV. STEADY-STATE CHARACTERIZATION OF THERAPEUTIC DOSE RANGE

As we investigate the therapeutic window of a NCE in man, the therapeutic dose range must be representative of pharmacologic and physiologic steady state. That is, the treatment should achieve pharmacokinetic as well as pharmacodynamic steady state and the physiological compensatory responses to the treatment should also be at steady state. Consideration of this steady-state condition is recognition that most, if not all, pathology represents perturbations of a multiplicity of physiologic balances.

More specifically, pathology actually represents a condition whereby compensatory mechanisms, which interact to maintain the physiologic balances within a "normal" range, can not adequately offset some perturbation to the normally balanced physiology. As we discuss in other chapters, chronic diseases are smaller persistent perturbations to normal physiology while acute diseases represent larger, more abrupt imbalances. In the context of this array of interacting and compensating physiologic balances, pharmacologic interventions are merely another influence in the system. Hopefully, these pharmacotherapies are helping to restore the normal balances. We must be mindful, however, that (1) the compensatory mechanisms may also respond to the therapy and (2) the therapy can overcome balanced physiology in another direction and thereby engender another perturbation by another mechanism. Also, establishing the new steady state which includes the pharmacotherapy may require considerable time. Further, the new steady state may be a less stable state than the pretreatment state. Consequently, the therapeutic dose range requires pharmacologic response to be determined after pharmacologic and physiologic steady state is attained. Attainment of steady state is probably most easily assessed by repeated measurements to assure that the patient is at steady state.

V. OPTIMAL BENEFIT/RISK PROFILE

Identification of a therapeutic dose range establishes that the NCE has some clinical utility and should be approvable based on demonstrated benefits that exceed risks in the clinical pharmacology evaluations during Phases I and II. In addition, the experience gained at this point makes it rational to proceed with larger studies in a broader sample of the target patient population. The principal questions that remain concern (1) establishing a reasonably precise quantification of the benefits and risks associated with therapy and (2) identifying the appropriate, hopefully near optimal, clinical use and patient population for this NCE. The clinically useful dose range will be defined by the experience gained from larger clinical trials involving a broad sample of the target patient population. The low end of the therapeutic dose range is likely to have the largest benefit/risk ratio since the risk factor should be low even for compounds that have fairly small separation between the efficacy and toxicity dose-response curves. However, the low end of the clinically useful dose range must have sufficient pharmacologic activity to represent a meaningful benefit to the patient. The lowest clinically useful dose will result from considering both the pharmacologic activity and the required clinical efficacy in the target patient population. Clinical experience will dictate this required activity. Often, 20% of the maximum achievable pharmacologic effect is a useful first approximation for the lowest clinically useful dose. This dose should produce a clinically useful pharmacologic effect in a significant portion of the patient population (e.g., 20–30%).

Larger patient experience will also increase the likelihood of detecting more subtle, less frequent pharmacologic effects (both desirable and undesirable) [11,13]. Depending upon the total patient experience, the lower limits of detection will approach 0.3–1% for a development program involving about 2,000 patients [11,13,14]. Programs involving 10,000 patients may be sensitive to drug-associated effects in the 0.1% range [11,13,14]. Obviously, there is little interest in therapeutic effects that small, but adverse events at that frequency may be important if they are serious or catastrophic. Of course, the difficulty here lies in identifying trends based on few events. For example, even in a 10,000 patient program an adverse event occurring at 0.1% would represent only 10 events. The 95% confidence interval includes 3–16 events. For most disease populations, such frequencies may not be obviously different from the background frequency of similar events in such patient populations [13,14]. To further complicate detection of infrequent events, it is also likely that the patient population studied in these late phase clinical trials will be a somewhat skewed sample compared with the population that will be treated after the drug is approved. Thus, the patient subpopulations that may be inadequately or inappropriately treated with some doses of the NCE will be difficult to detect by the current standards for the benefit/risk assessment and the current industry-supported trend to seek the broadest labeling possible for their NCEs [11]. In the final analysis, the current trend toward increasing sizes of Phase III programs [15] is probably accomplishing a small fraction of the anticipated gain because of our relatively poor ability to understand the variability among specific patient subpopulations at risk based on a study of the broadly defined target patient population.

VI. POPULATION VARIABILITY

It is very rare to find a patient population that is approximately homogeneous within the realm of human disease. Even in genetic diseases, which are considered to have specific, clearly defined etiologies, there is variability among individuals in terms of the progression of severity and sequelae of their disease (e.g., juvenile diabetes mellitus). It is also apparent that there is pharmacologic variability among patients. Some of this variability is related to subpopulations within a particular disease population. Patients with hypertension represent a well characterized example of a population that is very diverse, both in terms of the large variability of the disease and the variability of its responsiveness to pharmacotherapy

[16]. The range of the disease is well-documented from mild to moderate to severe. The medical community has even developed different therapeutic paradigms for these different categories of patients [16]. In addition, some patient subpopulations respond differently to the numerous therapies available to treat hypertension [16]. For example, black hypertensives are considered more responsive than white patients to thiazide-type diuretics [16]. Also interesting is the fact that doses of these thiazide-type diuretics used in practice have decreased significantly since their original approvals [16–18]. Neither racial differences nor apparent differences in the dose-response curves across the breadth of the hypertensive population were issues considered when these compounds were evaluated during the IND process. In fact, efficacy of the lower doses currently in use was unaddressed until it became apparent that at least some patients with relatively mild disease displayed serious untoward effects (e.g., electrolyte alterations) induced by long-term therapy with thiazide-type diuretics at doses above the minimum effective dose. It is fair to say that these long-term safety concerns for some subpopulations of the hypertensive population were unappreciated for many years after the original approvals of these drugs [19].

Armed with the recognition that the dose-response relationships and consequently the benefit/risk profiles may be sufficiently different among the subpopulations of various diseases, it is important that drug development programs address the issue of the most appropriate use of a given therapy across the target patient subpopulations. It is possible to address this issue in at least two ways. One method is to take advantage of the diversity among patients in the larger clinical trials and then exploit analyses that can facilitate an understanding of the differences occurring among the various subgroups. The other approach is to identify several clearly different patient subpopulations and determine the differences in their dose-response curves for efficacy and toxicity of the NCE. An understanding of the variation in response as a function of dose and variation in dose needed to achieve a given level of response will be required since it cannot be assumed that the various subpopulations will merely be represented by parallel dose-response curves. Rather, the family of dose-response curves may spread along both the dose-axis and response-axis with a variety of slopes, minima, and maxima. The variation in these curves is variability in responsiveness, beyond variability in measurement.

VII. SUMMARY

Thorough clinical characterization of the dose-response relationships for a NCE is an essential precursor to subsequent clinical studies in man. The approach outlined here is progressive. Initial work is directed toward determination of the investigational dose range (i.e., maximum no-effect dose to maximum tolerated dose). Then, a narrower portion is determined as the therapeutic dose range (i.e., minimum effective dose to maximum therapeutic dose). Knowledge of these dose ranges provides a framework for logical and systematic entry into expanded clinical trials.

REFERENCES

1. Food and Drug Administration. *General Considerations for the Clinical Evaluation of Drugs.* Washington, D.C.: U.S. Government Printing Office, September, 1977.
2. Title 21, *Code of Federal Regulations*, article 312.21.
3. Wardell WM. Scientific criteria and methods for drug assessment: requirements in the United States of America. In: *Drug Assessment: Criteria and Methods* (Bowers JZ, Velo GP, eds.). New York: Elsevier, 1979, pp. 91–100.
4. Cato AE. The challenge of the clinical development of drugs. In: *Clinical Drug Trials and Tribulations* (Cato AE, ed.). New York: Marcel Dekker, Inc., 1988, Chapter 1, pp. 1–16.
5. Cocchetto DM, Nardi RV. Challenges to maintaining continuity through expanded clinical trials and the approval period. In: *Clinical Drug Trials and Tribulations* (Cato AE, ed.). New York: Marcel Dekker, Inc., 1988, Chapter 14, pp. 253–274.
6. Spilker B, Cuatrecasas P. *Inside the Drug Industry.* Barcelona, Spain: Prous Science, 1989.
7. Geller NL. Design of phase I and II clinical trials in cancer: a statistician's view. *Cancer Investigation 2*: 483–491 (1984).
8. Guyatt G, Sackett D, Taylor DW, Chong J, Roberts R, Pugsley S. Determining optimal therapy—randomized trials in individual patients. *N. Engl. J. Med. 314*: 889–892 (1986).
9. Stolley PD, Strom BL. Sample size calculations for clinical pharmacology studies. *Clin. Pharmacol. Ther. 43*: 489–490 (1986).
10. Turri M, Stein G. The determination of practically useful doses of new drugs: some methodological considerations. *Statistics in Medicine 5*: 449–457 (1986).
11. Cocchetto DM, Nardi RV. Benefit-risk assessment of investigational drugs: current methodology, limitations and alternative approaches. *Pharmacotherapy 6*: 286–303 (1986).
12. Nardi RV, Cocchetto DM. Achievement of continuity and research equity in clinical drug development. *J. Clin. Res. Drug Development 1*: 153–165 (1987).
13. Jick H. Discovery of drug-induced illness. *N. Engl. J. Med. 296*: 481–485 (1977).
14. Jick H, Walker AM, Spriet-Pourra C. Postmarketing follow-up. *JAMA 242*: 2310–2314 (1979).
15. Jacob L, Carey R. A geocentric approach to sponsor conducted clinical trials. *J. Clin. Res. Drug Development 2*: 115–124 (1988).
16. 1988 Joint National Committee. The 1988 report of the Joint National Com-

mittee on detection, evaluation, and treatment of high blood pressure. *Arch. Intern. Med. 148*: 1023–1038 (1988).

17. The Joint National Committee on Detection, Evaluation and Treatment of High Blood Pressure. The 1980 report of the Joint National Committee on detection, evaluation and treatment of high blood pressure. *Arch. Intern. Med. 140*: 1280–1285 (1980).

18. The Joint National Committee on Detection, Evaluation and Treatment of High Blood Pressure. The 1984 report of the Joint National Committee on detection, evaluation and treatment of high blood pressure. *Arch. Intern. Med. 144*: 1045–1057 (1984).

19. Birkenhager WH, Solomon RJ, Wills MR, editors. Symposium on Electrolyte Disturbances and Cardiac Risks. *Drugs 28* (Suppl. 1): 1–199 (1984).

5

The Sliding Scale of Benefit/Risk Assessment

> For extreme diseases, extreme methods of cure, as to restriction, are most suitable.
>
> *Hippocrates*

I. INTRODUCTION

Several previous chapters have emphasized that benefit/risk assessment must be the focus of all drug development projects. Every project must begin to develop the benefit/risk assessment from the first time the new chemical entity is evaluated for its pharmacologic activity.

Benefit is defined as the pharmacotherapy-related reduction in disease-associated morbidity and mortality. Risk is defined as the increase in non-disease associated adverse events or drug-induced illnesses that are associated with pharmacotherapy. Approval and prescription availability of a new drug can only follow demonstration that the benefits of therapy exceed the risks, as required by federal regulation:

> An integrated summary of the benefits and risks of the drug, including a discussion of why the benefits exceed the risks under the conditions stated in the labeling. [1]

In disease terms, this means that the reduction in disease-associated morbidity and mortality must be greater than the increase in drug-associated risks. Of course, the total risk to patients is the composite of drug-associated risk plus the risk of residual disease-associated morbidity and mortality (i.e., that remaining despite pharmacotherapy). It is preferable to develop drugs such that this total risk is less than the drug-associated reduction in disease-associated morbidity and mortality.

As we discussed in previous chapters, benefit is dictated in large measure by the type of disease (acute, episodic, or chronic). Similarly, the disease is the predominant determinant of the acceptable level of risk associated with pharmacotherapy. The fact that the disease is the principal determinant of both achievable benefit and acceptable risk establishes the first of two benefit/risk sliding scales which must be addressed in planning and execution of a drug development project. One sliding scale is defined by the disease and a second sliding scale is defined by the patient subpopulation.

The major focus of this chapter will be the latter benefit/risk assessment sliding scale. It relates to the graded severity associated with many diseases, particularly episodic and chronic diseases, in various patient subpopulations. This particular benefit/risk assessment is sometimes ignored in drug development projects. This is unfortunate since it is the scale that may reflect the labeling needed to identify those patients likely to benefit most from new therapies and, even more importantly, identify those patients who are not good candidates for this particular therapy due to excessive risk with minimal benefit. Unfortunately, the physician in practice often conducts this type of benefit/risk assessment through "trial and error" via comparative assessment of various alternative treatments in individual patients [2,3]. An important consideration in development of any drug is the need for careful definition of appropriate patient candidates for the new drug. It will become imperative to understand the appropriate use of new drugs in sub-populations of patients with various diseases. This understanding will grow as medical science continues to improve its ability to identify and understand the natural history of disease processes, as well as expand our knowledge of the underlying physiologic mechanisms that change over time with advancing disease. We will illustrate some of these issues with examples in sections that follow.

II. SLIDING SCALE OF DISEASE-DICTATED BENEFIT AND RISK

It is easily understood that the more severe a disease, the higher the level of drug-associated risk that will be acceptable. This is simply the result of the fact that a therapy which ameliorates the effects of a life-threatening disease has such a large benefit that larger drug-associated risks can be tolerated in a beneficial drug. On the contrary, a self-limited acute disease with limited morbidity and no mortality serves as a setting where new drugs must have low drug-associated risk. This scale can be illustrated with a few examples based on the disease classification used in previous chapters.

A. Acute Disease

1. Myocardial Infarction

Consider a rather severe acute disease, myocardial infarction. Obviously, a myocardial infarction represents rather severe pathology in terms of its morbidity and mortality consequences. Both the immediate and long-term sequelae of this disease dictate that physicians undertake measures that primarily focus on preservation of life and secondarily focus on maximum preservation of myocardial function. In this setting, bypass surgery has become one of the possible interventions, even in the very early stages following onset of a myocardial infarction. Similarly, thrombolytic therapy with either streptokinase, tissue plasminogen activator (TPA), or anistreplase have acceptable benefit/risk profiles, even though 10-15% of patients experience some type of bleeding with thrombolytic drugs [4]. Intracranial hemorrhage, a potentially serious type of hemorrhage in such patients, has been reported at 0.4% frequency with up to 100 mg doses of TPA and 0.57% frequency with standard doses of anistreplase [4]. In the context of the high risks attendant to an untreated myocardial infarction, greater frequencies of drug-related adverse events can be acceptable.

Myocardial infarction is also associated with a high frequency of life-threatening arrhythmias. Aggressive anti-arrhythmic therapy is often used to treat patients in the early stages of a myocardial infarction and after infarction. However, most anti-arrhythmic drugs have narrow therapeutic windows and, in many cases, may themselves be arrhythmogenic in some concentrations. Similarly, beta-blockers have both benefits and risks. Beta-blockers have been shown to reduce the risk of reinfarction in the early stages following an initial myocardial infarction. However, beta-blockers carry the risk of inducing cardiac failure. Thus, the pattern emerging in this acute severe disease is that various therapies (including surgery, thrombolysis, antiarrhythmics, and beta-blockers) having substantial attendant risks are acceptable interventions in the context of a severe life-threatening disease such as a myocardial infarction.

Similar considerations apply in the case of bacterial meningitis. Drugs that would be acceptable treatments include some antibiotics that have a clear risk of some neurological damage and even some permanent or transient renal dysfunction. In this and other severe acute diseases, transient subjective complaints are of little consequence or consideration in defining the acceptable level of drug-associated risk. Reversible major organ system dysfunction (such as renal impairment) may also be acceptable in this setting, provided that it can be managed and does not increase the morbidity and mortality associated with the disease itself. Finally, irreversible major organ system dysfunction (e.g., ototoxicity) may also be tolerable provided that its long-term sequelae are consistent with life. Thus, in treating severe acute diseases, it can be acceptable to induce a drug-associated, manageable, chronic pathology in order to obtain the benefit of reduced mortality.

2. The Common Cold

Contrast this severe disease setting with a mild or self-limited acute disease such as the common cold. While the relative morbidity of the common cold is low, it is significant and important to consider the common cold in light of its large economic consequences and high prevalence. The common cold is a self-limited disease which will generally subside in one to two weeks even if left untreated. The issue in selecting any therapy today is whether treatment can improve the patient's quality of life while the disease is active. Further, treatment may reduce the usually low potential for any sequelae of this viral infection. Obviously, any pharmacotherapy that would carry any long-term risk would be unacceptable. In fact, it is unacceptable to trade on a one-to-one basis the congestion and its associated discomfort for drug-associated complaints. Of course, there is some disease-associated fatigue since the disease itself interferes with sleep. However, drug-induced drowsiness will cause patients to avoid using certain drugs and consequently interfere with the attainment of any therapy-associated benefits. Thus, in this setting of an acute self-limited mild disease, the acceptable level of drug-associated risk is dramatically lower than the previous example (myocardial infarction), and is probably limited to some level of subjective complaint. The acceptable level of risk is considerably less than the magnitude of reduction in quality of life associated with the disease.

These examples illustrate the very broad range of morbidity and mortality of acute diseases. They also serve as good illustrations of the level of drug-associated risks that can be tolerated in these settings.

B. Chronic Disease

The range of morbidity and mortality associated with various chronic diseases is also quite large, although remarkably different when compared with acute diseases. Chronic diseases by their very nature are consistent with life in the short term, but they represent reduction in quality of life or shortening of life expectancy, or both in the long term. Thus, the morbidities of chronic diseases are quite high, while mortality is only evident in the long term.

1. Parkinson's Disease

Parkinson's Disease is a chronic disease which can be severe. In most patients, the disease is progressive in that the patient gradually develops, over a period of years, more and more clinical symptoms. These symptoms are the manifestations and sequelae of the neurodegenerative process that is the underlying pathology of this disease. At present, there are some therapies such as L-dopa, carbidopa, and selegiline that contribute to reduced morbidity and improved quality of life of these patients. However, the adverse reactions reported with such therapies range from nausea to dementia and psychotic episodes, as well as some dystonic and involuntary movements. While the incidence of these more severe neurological adverse reactions is relatively low, it is notable that the disease is considered severe enough in terms of its morbidity to tolerate other drug-induced central nervous system disorders.

2. Gastroesophageal Reflux Disease

Like Parkinsonism, gastroesophageal reflux disease (GERD) is chronic in nature and there is a progressive worsening of the disease for some patients. Principally, however, morbidity is the result of a reduction in quality of life related to symptoms of this disease. Here again, the etiology of the underlying disease is not well understood. Consequently, available therapies are principally directed toward improving the quality of life for the affected patient. In the United States, three prescription drugs are presently approved for treatment of this disease: metoclopramide, ranitidine, and omeprazole. Antacids are useful as over-the-counter medication for the heartburn associated with gastroesophageal reflux. It is notable that GERD is a quantitative departure from normal physiology in that gastroesophageal reflux occurs normally in healthy individuals, particularly following meals. For most persons, this retrograde movement of the gastric contents into the esophagus is either unnoticed or only very infrequently results in symptoms. Patients who suffer from GERD experience the associated symptoms frequently. Reducing this symptomatology is a major thrust of the drug therapies that are presently available. Ranitidine has been demonstrated to reduce the heartburn associated with GERD. Ranitidine has a very low therapy-associated risk as it is a member of a class of drugs that is recognized to be among the safest pharmacotherapies on the market. Consequently, H-2-antagonist therapy has become an accepted standard for treatment of the symptoms of GERD. The heartburn associated with GERD is also reduced by metoclopramide, although to a lesser degree since it is principally a prokinetic agent. However, use of metoclopramide in this disease setting is not very popular due to adverse reactions ranging from nausea to Parkinsonian symptoms to other CNS effects, including depression. Clearly, although the drug-associated risks are similar for metoclopramide (used for GERD) and L-dopa (used for Parkinson's Disease) in terms of their severity, the large differences in the severities of the diseases for which these drugs are indicated clearly dictates the much more limited drug-associated risk acceptable in GERD, i.e., a chronic disease which is largely self-limited. Frequent and severe adverse reactions to drugs are not acceptable in this setting.

It is notable that metoclopramide was the first drug approved for GERD in the United States and it is questionable whether or not it would be approved for this indication today. The absence of any proven effective therapies for GERD at the time of metoclopramide's approval made the greater risk with this drug acceptable. We will return to this issue of appropriate use of metoclopramide for GERD as an illustration of the second type of benefit/risk sliding scale. The place for omeprazole in this disease will also be addressed, although it is notable that currently the drug-associated risks of omeprazole for short-term use appear to be minimal. Definition of the drug-associated long-term risks of omeprazole remains an open question. Since GERD is a chronic disease and the approved therapies are only indicated for relatively short-term use, the whole issue of appropriate therapy actually remains open in terms of the achievable benefit. However, it is clear that the acceptable drug-associated risks in this disease setting will of necessity be very low since the disease has little if any mortality and only subjective morbidity relating to the quality of life of the patient.

3. Final Considerations for Chronic Disease

The examples have illustrated that the range of severities of chronic diseases is very broad, although very different from the range for acute diseases. However, several examples have illustrated the principle that the acceptable drug-associated risk is dictated by the magnitude of disease-associated morbidity and mortality. Chronic neurodegenerative diseases such as Parkinsonism or other chronic severe diseases such as congestive heart failure have a higher level of acceptable drug-associated risk. In diseases with lower levels of morbidity and mortality, such as GERD, drug-associated adverse reactions must approach inconsequential levels. Clearly, the level of acceptable therapy-associated risk in chronic disease is much less than the level of therapy-associated risk in severe, acute diseases. There is some willingness to exchange some degree of improvement in quality of life for a limited magnitude of drug-associated risk. However, the frequency of these therapy-associated risks must be lower than the frequency of the disease-associated morbid events that the drug combats. As we progress to mild chronic diseases (e.g., GERD), the level of acceptable drug-associated risks gets even lower. Episodic diseases such as duodenal ulcer disease or gastric ulcer disease have a pattern quite similar to the pattern that is associated with chronic disease therapies. This is the result of repeated uses of the therapy over a patient's lifetime. We have addressed some of the issues regarding long-term use of pharmacotherapy for episodic diseases in other chapters.

III. SLIDING SCALE FOR DIFFERENT PATIENT SUBPOPULATIONS

The type of disease (acute, episodic, or chronic) and the disease itself are instrumental in dictating the acceptable level of drug-associated risk. We must now turn our attention to an aspect of benefit/risk assessment that is beginning to have an impact on the approval process. It will become far more important in the future. We are speaking of the *sliding scale for different patient subpopulations with a given disease.* For example, consider the severity of hypertension across patients with mild to moderate to severe disease. Asthma is commonly divided into patient subpopulations with mild, moderate, or severe disease. Similarly, there is a range of severity for congestive heart failure and progressive severity of some neurodegenerative diseases. In principle, the range of severity establishes subpopulations of patients with any given disease, in much the same way that different diseases establish different patient populations. These subpopulations can be diverse enough to dictate very different strategies in the approach to therapy. Consequently, these subpopulations are also very different in terms of the type of drug development they can enable. As a simple example, consider that a potential new bronchodilator drug can only be shown to reduce asthma-associated hospitalizations in a patient subpopulation with sufficiently severe asthma to produce some measurable frequency of hospitalization. Clearly, this drug effect could not be seen in a subpopulation of patient with very mild asthma and no appreciable frequency of hospitalization.

Hypertension is an extraordinarily good example of a disease in which much effort has gone into evaluating and categorizing patients by severity of disease. This effort has gone so far as to dictate totally different approaches to the acute and long-term management of patients with severe hypertension as opposed to patients with mild hypertension. However, drug developers have not made a comparable effort to address what we have termed the sliding scale of benefit/risk within the disease. This issue will be illustrated with a few examples, but the principles are not different from those described in the preceding section. Namely, *the severity and chronicity of the disease dictates both the required benefits and the level of acceptable drug-associated risk.* The drug development community must begin to aggressively identify the appropriate target subpopulations to receive new pharmacotherapies in development. It is apparent that much of this process of identifying the appropriate target subpopulations for a new drug has been done by practicing physicians through trial and error after approval and marketing of the drug. The drug development community should strive to establish labeling for new chemical entities that will facilitate targeted use of these drugs. We will illustrate these issues through a discussion of several diseases that are broadly recognized as having the variability that dictates different approaches to different patient subpopulations.

A. Hypertension

1. Subpopulations of Patients

There can be little argument that elevated blood pressure is associated with significant morbidity and mortality. Morbidity is often manifested as sequelae of the disease. Mortality is associated with some of these sequelae such as myocardial infarction or stroke. It is also clear from some very old data that antihypertensive pharmacotherapy has been shown to reduce some disease-associated risks. This has led to a leap of faith that all persons with blood pressures exceeding some preselected level have a chronic disease and consequently will benefit from life-long administration of drugs that lower blood pressure below some established limit. It is notable that the ability of pharmacotherapy in hypertension to reduce morbidity and mortality was established in patients with relatively severe forms of the disease, namely, diastolic blood pressures exceeding 115 mm Hg and 105 mm Hg in respective trials [5-7]. It has also become apparent that lower levels of blood pressure, namely, those exceeding 90 mm Hg diastolic or 140 mm Hg systolic have some associated morbidity and mortality. However, the series of studies that have been performed worldwide to evaluate treatment of mild hypertension provide ample evidence that the benefits of therapy are not nearly so sweepingly distributed as the dogma would lead one to believe [8-13].

The numerous commentaries on clinical trials on mild hypertension and the clinical treatment of mild hypertension document the controversy that exists in this area [14-19]. The data indicate that lowering blood pressure in patients with mild hypertension provides some quantitatively small benefit to this population of patients. This relatively smaller benefit is in sharp contrast to the larger therapeutic benefits observed in the previously mentioned treatment trials on more severe hypertension [5]. These small therapeutic benefits imply that the disease-associated risks in this population are small. This may arise for one of two reasons: first, each patient may have a very small risk associated with the elevation in blood pressure; second, and perhaps more likely, the patients who are actually at risk with these low elevations of blood pressure are a very small proportion of the total patients who are found to have blood pressures in the range for "mild" hypertension. Thus, aggressive therapy to lower blood pressure in the whole population of mildly hypertensive patients may provide little if any benefit to the majority of the recipients. While there certainly will be some patients who benefit from the therapy, many may only incur the drug-associated risks. This seems an inappropriate approach since some of these risks remain poorly defined.

2. Pathological Hypertension versus Incidental Hypertension

Further consideration of appropriate therapy for hypertension must consider the reports on placebo responders and patients who remain normotensive after discontinuation of medications. In the Australian trial, 48% of placebo-treated patients who were diagnosed as having blood pressures in the mild hypertension range had normal blood pressure at 3 years after enrollment in the trial [10,20]. In the Medical Research Council trial in the United Kingdom, similar findings were reported after 5 years of placebo therapy. The lability of blood pressure is well documented and clearly in both of these trials, as well as others, many patients identified as having a pathological departure from normal blood pressure may merely have labile, incidental high blood pressures that do not reflect pathology. Thus, these data suggest that a large portion of the patients receiving therapy for mild hypertension are actually receiving needless therapy.

These findings contributed to the necessity to perform therapy-withdrawal trials to confirm hypotensive effects of drugs via demonstrating return to hypertension after cessation of antihypertensive treatment. A number of these trials have found that substantial portions of patients assessed as having hypertension and requiring pharmacotherapy in fact remain normotensive for long periods of time after withdrawal of active antihypertensive therapy [21]. The inescapable conclusion from these data is that only a small portion of the patients who have elevated blood pressures in the mild hypertension range actually have the risks associated with disease and require long-term treatment.

Despite these data, the disease-associated risks of hypertension (i.e., risk of sudden cardiac death, myocardial infarction, and stroke) even in a small percentage of patients and the high prevalence of the disease have led the medical community to recommend treatment of mild hypertension. This direction would have little if any negative consequence if it were clear that the drug-associated risks of treating patients with mildly elevated blood pressures were negligible. Unfortunately, the data do not permit this conclusion. Needless pharmacotherapy is indeed a concern in view of the adverse events and drug-induced illnesses observed in hypertension trials. In some trials, some analyses suggest a numerical advantage for the placebo-treated control patients in terms of non-cardiovascular deaths [12,13] and sudden cardiac deaths in one trial [22]. It is impossible with the present data to determine whether some of the morbidity and mortality in these patients resulted from drugs that produced a pathological alteration of what was actually normal physiology for that patient.

3. Considerations for Studies of Antihypertensive Drugs

The drug development problem arises from the fact that the majority of hypertensive patients are in the category identified as mild hypertension. Also, the majority of patients enrolled in clinical trials on antihypertensive drugs have mild hypertension. It is clear that we can demonstrate the blood pressure lowering capabilities of antihypertensive therapies in this population of patients. However, it is an extraordinarily large leap of faith to conclude that lowering of blood pressure in this population of patients is equivalent to reducing the associated morbidity and mortality of hypertension. Blood pressure lowering is the gold standard for development of antihypertensive therapies. However, it is becoming increasingly clear that not all patients whose blood pressure is lowered experience therapy-associated benefits. That is, there is clearly a difference between the pharmacologic effects of a new chemical entity and the reduction in disease-associated morbidity. Consequently, most typical large Phase III multicenter trials conducted to document blood pressure lowering in patients with "hypertension" are really only demonstrating the pharmacologic activity of the new chemical entity. The studies do identify the untoward pharmacologic effects of the compound. The problem appears to lie in determining the distributions of therapeutic benefits and drug-associated risks. If it happens that the patients who are experiencing the untoward effects of these therapies are also receiving little or no benefit from these therapies, such patients represent a subpopulation who should be excluded from receiving this therapy.

An even greater controversy is the unknown effects of long-term antihypertensive therapy. Clinical trials in mild hypertension have documented that an untoward consequence of long-term diuretic therapy is increased likelihood of myocardial infarction. These consequences were unappreciated from the drug development trials that were performed in order to get some of these drugs approved. The emerging data on the effect of beta-blockers on lipid metabolism also suggest that we may be fixing one problem and creating another to the extent that the net effect may really have little therapeutic benefit for the patients. Since hypertension only has long-term disease-associated morbidity and mortality, we must become particularly sensitive to the issue of long-term therapy-associated risks. It may be possible to develop drugs which have few, if any, biochemical or physiologic effects other than reduction of blood pressure. Even if successful, we will be left with addressing the issue of whether blood pressure reduction in a patient who really does not have a pathologic elevation in blood pressure may have untoward consequences for that patient.

Hypertension is a particularly good illustration of the necessity to identify appropriate patients to receive therapy. This is an important issue even if one were able to develop a magic bullet which only lowered blood pressure and had no other physiologic effects. The drug development community has a stake in understanding these issues. It is incumbent upon the industry, FDA, and physicians to develop approaches to address these very important problems of administering appropriate antihypertensive therapy to the appropriate population of patients.

B.   Gastroesophageal Reflux Disease

GERD currently has three prescription therapies and some over-the-counter therapies that are approved for its treatment in the United States. It is interesting to note that the available therapies are separable by the severity of disease that they are appropriate for treating. In the United States, metoclopramide was the first prescription drug approved for GERD. As discussed above, this therapy has some significant side effects which have relegated it to use in a small subpopulation of patients with GERD. Current medical practice dictates that this compound is almost never used in the absence of failure of other therapies to control the symptoms of this disease.

Omeprazole was recently approved in the U.S. and is the newest compound for treatment of GERD. It is targeted at patients with very severe manifestations of GERD, particularly those patients with endoscopic evidence of esophagitis that includes erosive lesions and severe inflammatory lesions. Omeprazole is also quite effective for relief of symptoms (e.g., heartburn) associated with reflux disease.

Ranitidine is the only H-2-antagonist approved for treatment of GERD, although physicians commonly use all of the H-2-antagonists for this disease. Other H-2-antagonists will probably be approved for treatment of GERD in the near future. As a class of compounds, H-2-antagonists are effective in suppressing the heartburn associated with GERD. They are somewhat less dramatically effective for treating endoscopic esophagitis and the erosive and inflammatory lesions associated with severe GERD.

Consequently, the H-2-antagonists are broadly useful in the subpopulation of patients with mild to moderate GERD. Such a gradation of severity for reflux disease is consistent with the fact that GERD is associated with a quantitative increase from the normal amount of gastroesophageal reflux that occurs in healthy adults. Consequently, mild-to-moderate reflux disease includes patients who are closer to normal and may range to patients who have only mild or very infrequent esophageal mucosal damage.

Over-the-counter antacids represent a means to control some symptoms of GERD. That is, after symptoms have begun, antacid therapy can facilitate relief of symptoms. It is notable that symptoms are not always linked temporally to the actual reflux event. It may be that the heartburn symptoms actually occur only after significant damage to esophageal tissue has been done. Therefore, antacid therapy for patients who have relatively frequent heartburn is probably analogous to remembering to close the barn door after the horse got out. For patients with relatively infrequent symptoms of heartburn, however, antacids represent a means for relief, but they probably do not represent a means to control the underlying pathology.

While there appears to be a fairly impressive and broad armamentarium for treatment of GERD, none of these therapies are indicated for treatment lasting longer than a few weeks to a few months. None of these therapies have been studied for long-term management of this chronic disease. Further, the etiology of this disease is not well understood; the clinical manifestations of GERD may result from a multitude of factors that interact to produce or permit the disease. Since many patients need long-term therapy, potentially life-long therapy, it is indeed a glaring hole in the drug development efforts to have therapies identified only for short-term use in this disease setting. Another deficiency is our lack of knowledge about whether patients move from one level of disease-associated morbidity to a lower level of disease-associated morbidity as a result of drug therapy. For example, are patients who receive omeprazole to facilitate healing of their esophageal mucosa then able to undergo long-term therapy with an H-2-antagonist? If the answer is yes, we must then address the issue of what are the consequences of long-term therapy in this subpopulation of patients who have experienced severe manifestations of this disease. Yet another question is whether it is possible to intervene in milder stages of GERD and maintain patients in a relatively mild phase of the disease without running the risk of ultimately having patients progress to more severe manifestations. Further, if we treat patients with mild disease with very powerful agents such as a proton pump inhibitor, are these patients at any long-term risk associated with complete abrogation of normal physiologic secretions into the GI tract?

Again, the example of GERD emphasizes the importance of identifying appropriate subpopulations to receive each particular new drug. This is an extraordinarily important issue both for the drugs that presently exist to treat this disease and for those that will be developed in the future. Our relative naivete about the disease itself makes it more important for us to be conservative in terms of applying pharmacotherapies without a complete understanding of the therapy-associated risks.

C. Thrombolytic Therapy for Myocardial Infarction

The controversy prior to approval of tissue plasminogen activator (TPA) for thrombolytic therapy in myocardial infarction is another illustration of the importance of understanding the appropriate subpopulations for whom new pharmacotherapies are most judiciously used. Unfortunately for the sponsor, FDA, and patients, the drug development process was not able to identify any broadly accepted advantage of TPA over other thrombolytic therapies. In fact, it was not clear initially whether TPA had the same benefits as streptokinase. Nor was it clear whether adverse events associated with TPA were any different in either kind or frequency from the adverse events associated with streptokinase. Consequently, the high expectations that accompanied introduction of TPA into clinical trials in the U.S. were unmet by the data filed with FDA to seek approval for the compound. While TPA may have been developed quickly, the result has been a compound that is far below expectations. Among the issues that went unaddressed in the TPA submission was whether it identified a group of patients who was clearly in need of this therapy relative to the potential benefits from other therapies. Both urokinase and streptokinase were approved before TPA. On approval, TPA was just another thrombolytic agent with no patient subpopulation having unique benefit from the therapy and no patient subpopulation having an unique safety advantage compared with other thrombolytic therapies. It may be that over time the quality of TPA and its advantage as a thrombotic therapy relative to other available thrombolytic therapies will be proven. However, the present data leave this an open question. The benefit/risk profile of TPA does not appear to be dramatically different from other thrombolytic therapies. It is not clear whether patients with relatively mild infarction, i.e., those involving small regions of the myocardium, benefit more from one of the available thrombolytic therapies compared with patients with larger infarcted regions. Similarly, it is not clear whether patients with relatively large areas of ischemia may benefit uniquely from one particular thrombolytic therapy. It is also not clear if the treatment failures from one therapy might in fact be treatment successes on another therapy. All of these questions are addressable in the context of a drug development program. In fact, the data to answer some of the questions may already exist as secondary information in studies already done.

D. NSAID-Induced Ulcers

One very good example of a drug that is currently approved as a result of identifying a unique patient population for whom this therapy had some advantage is misoprostol, the prostaglandin analogue. The original NDA for this drug was submitted to the agency for treatment of duodenal ulcer disease. While it was more effective than placebo, it was not clear that this drug offered any more benefit relative to other available antiulcer therapies. More importantly, misoprostol had a major associated risk as an abortifacient. This risk rendered the compound unapprovable because clearly the benefit could not outweigh this risk in the setting of duodenal ulcer disease. Subsequently, this compound was shown to be effective for the prevention and treatment of NSAID-induced gastric ulcers. In this respect, this compound was unique among all of the anti-ulcer compounds at least according to the data available to FDA at the time of approval. Consequently, misoprostol was approved for this use. The issue that still remains with the approval of this compound is who among this population of patients really benefits from its use. It is fairly clear from the literature that not all patients receiving NSAIDS, including aspirin, will experience gastrointestinal distress or ulceration as a result of the therapy. Thus, administration of misoprostol to the population of patients receiving NSAID therapy is really only justifiable if there are no substantial attendant risks of receiving this therapy or if a patient subgroup has greater probability of developing an NSAID-induced ulcer. Clearly, the former is not true for misoprostol and, therefore, its use has been restricted to subpopulations with enhanced probability of an NSAID-induced ulcer.

IV. TREATMENT FAILURES

An issue that is not commonly addressed in conventional drug development programs is identification of the characteristics of patients who are highly unlikely to respond to the new drug. This is a population of patients for whom therapy provides no benefit. These patients represent a subpopulation in every drug development program; they incur risks and no benefit. Similar patients receive the new drug after approval and they receive no benefit and incur risks.

Follow-up of treatment failures is an issue that must be addressed if we are to understand how the sliding scale of benefit/risk fits into the development of drugs for a specific disease. Clearly, treatment failures have the lowest possible benefit/risk ratio. The issue of identifying the various non-responsive subpopulations is indeed one that must be addressed in the next decade of drug development.

V. SUMMARY

Several examples have been used to impart some operational guidance regarding the sliding scale assessment of benefit and risk. The two fundamental messages are straightforward. First, the severity and chronicity of the disease are the primary determinants of both the required benefit and the level of acceptable drug-associated risk. In discussing metoclopramide as the first drug approved for treatment of GERD, we alluded to one secondary determinant of the level of acceptable benefit and risk. That is, the notion that the benefit/risk ratio of an approved drug (for the same indication as a new investigational drug) usually sets a standard for the minimum benefit/risk ratio that is acceptable for subsequent proposed new drugs for the disease. Of course, this minimum acceptable benefit/risk ratio tends to increase as more drugs are approved for the indication.

The second fundamental message is that each overall population of patients with a particular disease must be fractionated so that the drug developer can describe the characteristics of each specific patient subpopulation that attains a favorable benefit/risk ratio from the drug, as well as describe those patient subpopulations who should not receive the drug in view of their known disfavorable benefit/risk ratios. Operationally, separation of these various patient subpopulations can be difficult, but it is nonetheless essential.

REFERENCES

1. *Code of Federal Regulations*. Title 21, article 314.50(d)(5)viii. Washington, D.C.: U.S. Government Printing Office, p. 103, 1989.
2. Guyatt G, Sackett D, Taylor DW, Chong J, Roberts R, Pugsley S. Determining optimal therapy—randomized trials in individual patients. *N. Engl. J. Med. 314*: 889–892 (1986).
3. Guyatt GH, Keller JL, Jaeschke R, Rosenbloom D, Adachi JD, Newhouse MT. The n-of-1 randomized controlled trial: clinical usefulness. Our three-year experience. *Ann. Intern. Med. 112*: 293–299 (1990).
4. *1990 Physicians' Desk Reference*. Oradell, NJ: Medical Economics Co., 44th Edition, 1990.
5. Veterans Administration Cooperative Study Group on Antihypertensive Agents. Effects of treatment on morbidity in hypertension. Results in patients

with diastolic blood pressures averaging 115–129 mm Hg. *JAMA 202*: 1028–1034 (1967).

6. Veterans Administration Cooperative Study Group on Antihypertensive Agents. Effects of treatment on morbidity in hypertension. II. Results in patients with diastolic blood pressure averaging 90 through 114 mm Hg. *JAMA 213*: 1143–1152 (1970).

7. Veterans Administration Cooperative Study Group on Antihypertensive Agents. Effects of treatment on morbidity and mortality. III. Influence of age, diastolic pressure, and prior cardiovascular disease; further analysis of side effects. *Circulation 45*: 991–1004 (1972).

8. Smith WM. Treatment of mild hypertension: results of a ten-year intervention trial. *Circ. Res. 40* (Suppl. I): I98–I105 (1977).

9. Hypertension Detection and Follow-Up Program Cooperative Group. Five-year findings of the Hypertension Detection and Follow-Up Program. I. Reduction in mortality of persons with high blood pressure, including mild hypertension. *JAMA 242*: 2562–2571 (1979).

10. The Management Committee. The Australian therapeutic trial in mild hypertension. *Lancet 1*: 1261–1267 (1980).

11. Helgeland A. Treatment of mild hypertension: a five year controlled drug trial. The Oslo study. *Amer. J. Med. 69*: 725–732 (1980).

12. Multiple Risk Factor Intervention Trial Research Group. Multiple Risk Factor Intervention Trial: risk factor changes and mortality results. *JAMA 248*: 1465–1477 (1982).

13. Medical Research Council Working Party. MRC trial of treatment of mild hypertension: principal results. *Brit. Med. J. 291*: 97–104 (1985).

14. Kaplan NM. Whom to treat: the dilemma of mild hypertension. *Amer. Heart J. 101*: 867–870 (1981).

15. Freis ED. Should mild hypertension be treated? *N. Engl. J. Med. 307*: 306–309 (1982).

16. W.H.O./I.S.H. Mild Hypertension Liasson Committee. Trials of the treatment of mild hypertension: an interim analysis. *Lancet 1*: 149–156 (1982).

17. Breckenridge A. Treating mild hypertension. *Brit. Med. J. 291*: 89–90 (1985).

18. Moser M, Gifford RW. Why less severe degrees of hypertension should be treated. *J. Hypertens. 3*: 437–447 (1985).

19. Ramsay LE. Mild hypertension: treat patients, not populations. *J. Hypertens. 3*: 449–455 (1985).

20. A Report by the Management Committee of the Australian herapeutic Trial in Mild Hypertension. Untreated mild hypertension. *Lancet 1*: 185–191 (1982).

21. Nardi RV. Commentary on "Prolonged normotension after abrupt withdrawal of terazosin treatment: implications for studies of the efficacy of antihypertensive drugs." *J. Clin. Res. Drug Development 1*: 301–305 (1987).

22. Sherwin R (for the MRFIT Research Group). Sudden death in men with increased risk of myocardial infarction: the MRFIT programme. *Drugs 28* (Suppl. 1): 46–53 (1984).

6

Treatment Use of Investigational Drugs: A Special Setting for Benefit/Risk Assessment

> It is not a case we are treating; it is a living,
> palpitating, alas, too often suffering fellow creature.
>
> *John Brown*

I. INTRODUCTION

Previous chapters have discussed concepts of clinical drug development, dose-response characterization, and benefit/risk assessment. We highlighted the importance of considering the various subpopulations of patients within the target disease population. For example, subpopulations of interest can be delineated by strata of severity of the target disease or different subpopulations can be defined by concomitant conditions (e.g., renal failure). In this chapter, we will consider two additional subpopulations, i.e., the subpopulation of patients who have failed all other therapies for their disease and the subpopulation of patients for whom there is no approved treatment. The ethical, medical, scientific, and regulatory issues concerning use of investigational drugs in these two subpopulations have led to special regulations and guidances, as well as considerable ongoing discussion among physicians, patients, FDA, sponsors, clinical drug developers, and legislators. We will describe and compare the current options for treatment use of investigational drugs.

In its broadest sense, treatment use of an investigational new drug is defined as provision of a supply of a specific investigational drug to a requesting physician/investigator for the expressed purpose of treating specific patients with a potentially responsive disease which has to date failed to respond to an adequate course of treatment with commercially available therapies. In general, diseases for which treatment use is sought are associated with either high morbidity (e.g., Alzheimer's disease or Gilles de la Tourette's syndrome) or high mortality (e.g., AIDS), or both. Treatment use is particularly important for promising investigational new drugs when no adequate therapy is approved for treatment of the disease in the United States.

There exist broad public acceptance and support from FDA for the concept of providing promising investigational new drugs to desperately ill patients as early as it is reasonable in the clinical drug development process [1,2]. Nonetheless, inappropriate treatment use of investigational drugs would be irresponsible by giving patients false hope and may be unsafe by worsening the original condition. These last two sentences summarize the dilemma of treatment use of investigational drugs.

Treatment use cases can comprise a meaningful addition to the knowledge base on a drug in clinical development. Treatment use of an investigational new drug can be implemented as early as Phase II of the clinical drug development process, as long as there exists reasonable evidence that the drug has a favorable benefit/risk ratio for the intended patients [2].

The FD&C Act requires that only drugs proven to be safe and effective and hence approved for use in the U.S. be administered as "treatments." However, the Act and certain regulations developed to implement the Act recognize selected circumstances in which an unapproved investigational new drug may have sufficient data to warrant its use as "treatment" for selected patients. Such treatment use of investigational drugs can occur via three mechanisms that are described in current final regulations: (1) Treatment IND regulations, (2) Subpart E regulations, or (3) Emergency Use regulations. This chapter will describe and compare each of these three approaches. In addition, two very recent methods of treatment use (parallel track mechanism and importation of drugs for personal use) are briefly described.

II. REGULATORY CONSIDERATIONS FOR A TREATMENT IND

The Food and Drug Administration issued final rules regarding Treatment INDs in 1987 [3]. These rules have been the subject of papers intended to inform the medical community about their provisions [2,4-6]. These regulations became effective for protocols and INDs submitted after June 22, 1987. The term "treatment use of investigational drugs" is founded in the Food, Drug, and Cosmetic Act and the subsequent regulations of the

IND rewrite since investigational drugs are not customarily described as "treatments" as their efficacy and safety have not yet been established [7]. However, the regulations effective June 22, 1987 provide for the use of certain investigational drugs as treatments under selected circumstances. A Treatment IND can be issued to a sponsor (e.g., a pharmaceutical company or the National Institutes of Health) or to an individual physician.

Treatment use of an investigational new drug shall be permitted under a treatment protocol or treatment IND if each of the following five conditions apply [3]:

1. The investigational new drug is intended to treat a serious or immediately life-threatening disease.
2. The investigational new drug is being studied in a controlled clinical trial for the serious or immediately life-threatening disease, or a very similar disease state,

   or

   such controlled clinical trials on the drug have been completed.
3. There is no comparable or satisfactory alternative drug or other therapy available to treat that stage of the disease in the intended patient population.
4. The sponsor of the controlled clinical trial is demonstrating due diligence to actively pursue marketing approval of the investigational new drug.
5. If the investigational new drug is intended to treat a serious disease, there must be sufficient evidence of the safety and effectiveness of the drug to support its proposed treatment use.

   or

   If the investigational new drug is intended to treat an immediately life-threatening disease, there must be sufficient evidence to provide a reasonable basis for concluding that the drug (a) may be effective for its intended treatment use in the intended patient population and (b) will not expose the intended patients to an unreasonable and significant additional risk of drug-associated illness or injury.

This last condition necessitates definitions of immediately life-threatening disease and serious disease. An *immediately life-threatening disease* is a stage of a disease associated with a reasonable likelihood that death will occur within a matter of months (generally, within 6 months) or in which premature death is likely without early treatment. Examples of such diseases are advanced congestive heart failure (New York Heart Association class IV), advanced cases of AIDS, bacterial endocarditis, metastatic refractory cancer, and far advanced emphysema [2,3]. A *serious disease* is a stage of a disease in which substantial morbidity is present, but in which premature death without early treatment or a high short-term mortality rate are not considerations. Examples of serious diseases are Alzheimer's disease, advanced multiple sclerosis, advanced Parkinson's disease, transient ischemic attacks, and some types of seizure disorders [2,3].

Given the specification of types of diseases and the conditions under which a Treatment IND shall be granted, it is clear that the ultimate standard for denying treatment use of a drug for an immediately life-threatening disease is insufficient evidence that the drug may be effective or insufficient evidence that the drug would not comprise an unreasonable, significant additional risk for the patient. For serious diseases, the ultimate standard for denying treatment use is more demanding, i.e., insufficient evidence of the safety and effectiveness of the drug. Application of these criteria by FDA to the early submissions for Treatment IND status has been described [8].

Interestingly, a properly initiated, ongoing protocol for treatment use of an investigational drug may be placed on clinical hold by FDA if any one of the previously cited five conditions becomes inapplicable. For example, if a comparable or satisfactory alternative drug or other therapy becomes available, the protocol for treatment use could be placed on clinical hold.

The conditions for treatment use are intended to make a promising investigational new drug (not yet approved for marketing for any use) available to desperately ill patients when there exists reasonable evidence to support the conclusion that the drug *may* be effective in these desperately ill patients and that the drug will *not* comprise an unreasonable, significant new risk for the patient. That is, there must be reasonable evidence to argue that a favorable benefit/risk ratio exists for the intended patients. In the commentary portion of the relevant regulations, FDA states its recognition of the different benefit/risk ratios that would be acceptable in different patient populations [3]. For example, a lower benefit/risk ratio would be more acceptable for treatment use of an investigational new drug for treatment of a patient with advanced AIDS (i.e., an immediately life-threatening disease) than for a patient with a serious, but not immediately life-threatening, disease.

A Treatment IND is subject to all of the provisions of the general IND process. Any treatment use of an investigational new drug requires the sponsor and investigator to comply with all of the provisions of the IND process, including assuring administration of the drug under the supervision of an investigator who is qualified by appropriate training and experience, monitoring by the sponsoring organization, granting of informed consent by the patient, review by an institutional review board, and timely reporting of adverse events. Treatment use of the drug under a treatment protocol (whether as an amendment to an existing IND or in a separate Treatment IND) may begin 30 days after the submission is received at FDA, unless disapproval is expressed by FDA. It remains to be assessed whether the application of these general IND regulations to the special case of a Treatment IND will, in practice, reduce the speed with which promising investigational drugs can reach patients or provide an appropriately cautious environment for treatment use of investigational drugs.

III. SUBPART E DESIGNATION

An interim rule for public comment was issued October 21, 1988 for Subpart E which appears as 21 CFR 312.80 [9]. Subpart E applies only to drugs intended to treat life-threatening and severely debilitating illnesses. This interim rule is intended to expedite marketing of significant new treatments and it is the logical partner of the 1987 regulations on Treatment INDs. The purpose of a Treatment IND is to provide a regulatory procedure through which promising investigational new drugs with limited evidence of safety and efficacy can be supplied for treatment of patients with serious or immediately life-threatening disease. Granting of a Treatment IND by FDA does not, in and of itself, indicate a greater or lesser likelihood of ultimate FDA approval of the drug for marketing, nor does it necessarily indicate establishment of a collaboration between FDA and the sponsor to assure that the sponsor's controlled clinical trials will meet the criteria of adequate and well-controlled as needed to support approval. The Subpart E regulations provide a regulatory means to fill the gap between the achievement of a Treatment IND (i.e., bringing the drug to individual patients during the IND stage) and achieving an approved, marketed product.

Subpart E describes a process of intensive and frequent exchanges between sponsor and FDA at both the pre-IND stage and the end of Phase I. The purpose of these exchanges is to interactively review and agree on the appropriate preclinical studies, Phase I studies, and Phase II clinical trials needed to collect sufficient data to prove safety and efficacy in a manner that can support approval of the drug, assuming the data are indeed supportive. This series of preclinical and clinical studies will be agreed to be appropriate in the sense of including rigorous prospective selection of suitable variables and therapeutic endpoints, acceptable unit dose and dosage regimen, reasonable duration of treatment, reasonable duration of monitoring of the patients for assessment of efficacy and safety, and attention to prospective monitoring of both short-term and long-term potential toxicitites of the drug. This aggressive approach of designing targeted Phase I and II studies with the possibility of supporting approval holds the promise of helping some drugs become available sooner for the treatment of life-threatening and severely debilitating illnesses. In the context of Subpart E, a life-threatening disease is a disease with a high likelihood of death unless the course of disease is interrupted and where survival is an endpoint of the clinical trial. A severely debilitating disease is defined in Subpart E as a disease causing major irreversible morbidity. The regulation encourages sponsors to consult FDA on applicability of these definitions to specific patient populations for specific investigational drugs.

A promising drug that successfully progresses through preclinical studies, Phase I, and Phase II may show favorable safety and efficacy results as early as an interim analysis of a Phase II study. When such favorable results are available, Subpart E states that FDA may ask the sponsor to submit a treatment protocol as described in the Treatment IND regulations (21 CFR 312.34). Such a protocol would be expected to be a means of supplying the drug to the target patient subpopulations until the NDA could be prepared, submitted, reviewed, and approved. Interestingly, the Subpart E regulations do *not* state any timeframe for review of such an NDA different from the timeframe applicable to any NDA for any other drug.

Johnstone [10] has raised interesting questions about the ultimate utilization of the Treatment IND and Subpart E regulations by sponsors. He questions whether sponsors will assume the added risk of investigational treatment use and, indeed, whether it is practical to pursue treatment use when such use must satisfy the full spectrum of IND regulations. Clearly, clinical trials conducted under Subpart E or a Treatment IND are subject to monitoring by the sponsor, IRB approval, informed consent, field auditing by FDA, and all other provisions of the IND regulations. Perhaps most importantly, Johnstone [10] wonders whether FDA will tend to keep a drug subject to a Treatment IND or Subpart E development off the market until all of the safety questions that arise in treatment use are resolved. In view of the lack of regulatory assurance of rapid review and approval of such programs, sponsors assume a risk from pursuing such programs. This risk must be balanced against the likelihoods of more rapid clinical drug development and earlier approval.

IV. EMERGENCY (COMPASSIONATE) USE

Compassionate treatment with an investigational new drug is a nonstandardized approach to therapy for patients with a potentially responsive, serious or life-threatening disease which has failed to respond to adequate courses of currently approved therapies. The nature of compassionate treatment necessitates that a physician/investigator make a decision to request use of a specific investigational drug for a specific patient and consequently that the pharmaceutical company also make a decision regarding supplying the drug on an individual drug and individual patient basis.

Pharmaceutical corporate sponsors of the development of new chemical entities may receive premarketing requests for compassionate use of certain investigational drugs. Since this type of request is widely recognized among practicing university-affiliated physicians and pharmaceutical companies, the paucity of published information on this topic is surprising. Rodel [11] published an abstract on the compassionate use protocol as a useful methodology for clinical research on enalapril maleate. Several brief news releases regarding compassionate use of various drugs have been published in trade journals of the pharmaceutical industry [12,13]. A full manuscript describing the experience of Burroughs Wellcome with Zidovudine has been published [14].

The existence of so-called "compassionate treatment INDs" is not recognized as such in the regulations. However, provision of an investigational new drug on such a compassionate, i.e., emergency use basis, has been accomodated by the IND rewrites (21 CFR 312.36, Emergency Use of an Investigational New Drug). In such cases, the regulations allow FDA to authorize shipment of the drug for a specified use prior to submission of the appropriate IND or amendment to the IND, provided that the appropriate submission is completed as soon as practical. This regulation is open-ended in the sense that it does not *a priori* restrict such emergency use to patients with serious or life-threatening diseases.

The regulations on emergency use of IND drugs do not define what constitutes an emergency, but Beers [15] reported that the devices policy would probably prove acceptable for drugs. For medical devices, an emergency is comprised of the following four features [16]:

1. A patient with a life-threatening condition or potential loss of a major bodily function.
2. A condition that requires immediate treatment.
3. No generally acceptable alternative treatment is available.
4. There is insufficient time to permit conventional procedures to be used to gain access to the investigational treatment.

Although review and approval by an IRB is preferred prior to use of the drug, the regulations allow emergency use without prior IRB approval as long as a report is submitted to the IRB within five working days of drug use (21 CFR 56.104c).

Appler [17] has recommended that treatment use under a compassionate IND, as well as treatment use under a Treatment IND, receive more comprehensive discussion in more public forums. There is no central registry available to physicians to disclose a list of drugs available under compassionate IND or Treatment IND. Institution of such a central list by FDA was suggested by Former FDA Chief Counsel Peter Barton Hutt [18]. He also suggested on February 16, 1988 at a joint FDA/AMA conference on Treatment INDs that an urgent need existed for practical information on how a physician can obtain a Treatment IND and who can be called for answers regarding investigational drugs for treatment use [18]. These suggestions were addressed by FDA Commissioner Young when he initiated in July 1988 a series of publications in the *Journal of the American Medical Association* on investigational drugs for treatment use [5,6].

The urgency and volume of compassionate treatment requests vary considerably. The urgency of these requests is determined by (1) the acute versus chronic nature of the disease process to be treated; (2) the goal of reducing either morbidity, mortality, or both; and (3) the existence of other approved or unapproved therapies. The volume of compassionate treatment requests is determined by:

1. The frequency of presentation of truly appropriate patient candidates
2. Availability of other therapy
3. The physician's willingness to use an investigational drug in view of the paperwork involved and, in most cases, little or no prior experience with the drug
4. The degree of physician awareness of the drug
5. The degree of acceptability of compassionate treatment to local institutional review boards
6. The sponsor's willingness to respond favorably to a compassionate request.

Requests for compassionate treatment of a life-threatening acute disease require intensive initial efforts due to the need to respond to each request within a few hours. The time required for a pharmaceutical company to respond to each of these requests is significant, as is the time required for close follow-up. In addition to the time required from the clinical research staff, secretarial support must be substantial, as is the support of pharmacy personnel to assure that clinical trial materials (e.g., drug, protocol, case report form, Clinical Investigator Brochure) are sent in the most rapid manner. For compassionate treatment of a chronic disease, a prospective commitment by the sponsor, investigator, and patient to longer-term data collection and monitoring must be present.

V. ADDITIONAL METHODS FOR TREATMENT USE OF INVESTIGATIONAL DRUGS

A. Parallel Track Mechanism

FDA will continue to work with physicians and patient advocacy groups to create new, controlled methods to make promising investigational new drugs available for treatment use. One such new, controlled method is the proposed policy on a parallel track mechanism for expanded availability of promising investigational drugs to patients with AIDS and HIV-related diseases [19]. This policy proposes a specific method by which the traditional controlled clinical trials (the conventional basis for approval of new drugs) can proceed, yet a concurrent group of studies (so-called parallel track studies) can be conducted (1) without a concurrent control group, (2) to provide the drug to a broader group of patients than can qualify for the controlled trials, and (3) to collect data on safety of the drug. This proposal is an example of the creative new approaches being demanded by the AIDS crisis, but it is reasonable to expect that the best of these new approaches will ultimately be used to enable expanded availability of other investigational drugs for other indications.

B. Importation of Unapproved Drugs for Personal Use

FDA recognizes that more Americans will purchase drug products abroad as international trade and world travel increase. Some of these products will not be approved for sale in the U.S. However, the *Regulatory Procedures Manual* encourages FDA personnel to consider a more permissive policy for certain importations of personal-use quantitites of drugs [20]. This relatively new provision has facilitated the efforts of some patients with AIDS to import personal-use quantities of certain drugs that are not approved for use in the U.S.

VI. CONSIDERATIONS IN THE DECISION TO PURSUE TREATMENT USE OF AN INVESTIGATIONAL DRUG

Treatment use of an investigational drug may be approached from the perspective of considering the advantages and disadvantages of pursuing this use. Table 1 lists several situations in which treatment use may be valuable to both the sponsor and the patient. These situations are atypical of the setting of conventional clinical drug development.

In some situations, requests for treatment use can not be considered (Table 2). The more common of these situations are inadequate drug supply

Table 1. Situations in which some form of treatment use of an investigational drug may be useful to patient and sponsor.

1. no pharmacotherapy or other therapy is currently available for cure, control, or palliation of the disease
2. the population of patients in the desired stage of the target disease (e.g., demonstrated unresponsive) is small in any one center
3. availability of highly effective and safe therapies may, in some settings, preclude assessment of an investigational drug in all but those patients who are demonstrated non-responders to available therapies
4. the prevalence of the target disease is low so as to preclude treatment of an acceptably large patient population in a conventional single center or multicenter clinical trial
5. need to study safety of the drug in a large number of patients with the target disease in the general medical care setting in a non-comparative study in a short period of time (e.g., zidovudine for patients with AIDS)
6. opportunity to characterize the patient population which fails to respond to one or more alternative therapies
7. initial evaluation of the efficacy and safety of different prototypical compounds in patients with a rapidly advancing disease for which there is no approved therapy

and exclusion of the patient due to some concurrent disorder or complication which would render use of the drug excessively hazardous to the patient. When none of the pre-emptive factors in Table 2 apply, the specific case must be considered to decide whether or not to pursue treatment use. Table 3 lists some common reasons for choosing not to pursue treatment use of an investigational drug.

Table 2. Situations in which some form of treatment use of an investigational drug can not be considered.

1. lack of approval by FDA for treatment use under the IND
2. inadequate supply of drug
3. lack of approval of institutional review board
4. lack of informed consent from patient
5. patient does not pass inclusion/exclusion criteria of treatment protocol (e.g., presence of a concurrent disorder or condition such as anuria or pregnancy that precludes use of the drug)
6. inability or unwillingness of physician to adhere to treatment and patient monitoring provisions of the treatment protocol
7. inadequate resources of sponsor preclude adequate monitoring in accordance with IND regulations

Table 3. Reasons to withhold an investigational drug from treatment use.

A. Administrative:
1. inadequate supply of drug
2. inadequate pharmacy personnel to prepare and ship drug
3. inadequate personnel and time for monitoring by the sponsor
4. adverse impact of treatment use on enrollment in controlled trials
5. unacceptable liability

B. Regulatory:
1. FDA does not endorse the approach for a specific drug
2. inexperienced investigators may not comply fully with regulations
3. lack of approval by an institutional review board
4. lack of informed consent
5. inadequate information on the patient provided by the investigator

C. Medical:
1. lack of reasonable evidence of efficacy of the drug
2. lack of reasonable evidence of safety of the drug
3. patient at end-stage of a chronic disease with high mortality rate
4. patient has not received an adequate trial of alternative drug therapies and other therapies
5. equivocal status of the diagnosis
6. pregnancy or childbearing potential without adequate contraceptive method

VII. INVESTIGATOR AND SPONSOR RESPONSIBILITIES

It is the responsibility of the investigator to limit applications for treatment use for an investigational drug to requests on behalf of patients who clearly have not responded to adequate courses of alternative therapies and have not progressed to the end stages of a fatal disease. A request also signifies the investigator's acceptance of his obligations as an investigator with respect to the guidelines and IND regulations pursuant to the FD&C Act [21,22]. In practice, some physicians fail to fulfill their obligations as investigators after having undertaken treatment use of an investigational drug. Given the urgency of caring for a patient with an immediately life-threatening disease, for example, some investigators contend that collecting only a portion of the necessary documentation (e.g., case report, consent form) should be adequate. This contention is clearly contrary to the regulations. In addition, such an approach diminishes the contribution of data from these patients to the overall benefit/risk profile of the new drug, as well as minimizing the application of important knowledge gained from treating one patient to decision making for the next patient.

In sponsoring a Treatment IND or responding to compassionate treatment requests, the corporate sponsor incurs obligations to the sponsor itself, the FDA, the requesting investigator, and the patient. These obligations are the same as those in any prospective clinical trial. However, the obligations of the sponsor to the specific investigator and patient are more pronounced in this setting of the diminished time frame for action. The investigator is seeking what he assesses as the only possibly effective therapy for his patient. The obligation to the patient is sometimes difficult to perceive for the sponsor, as a distant party, but it is easily imagined in terms of a similar situation with a former patient or a family member. The sponsor must make decisions based on the sponsor's responsibility as a member of the medical community. In some cases, this means supplying the investigational drug. In other cases, this means suggesting possible alternative therapies that have not yet been explored. Some alternative therapies may themselves be other investigational drugs. Admittedly, the adequacy of drug inventory can be the single largest problem in responding to these requests since full-scale manufacturing procedures and facilities will often not yet be developed while the drug is still in investigational Phase II or Phase III.

Interest in treatment use of an investigational drug tends to be greatest for diseases with no other therapy. Such interest tends to grow as soon as early evidence of efficacy emerges in Phase II. One example is the treatment of AIDS-related complex (ARC) and acquired immunodeficiency syndrome (AIDS) with one of the investigational drugs zidovudine [14,23] or isoprinosine [24]. Although the initial requests for such drugs preceded the availability of substantial evidence of efficacy from controlled clinical trials, the drugs represented a tangible hope to some patients and physicians. This hope is evident in one AIDS patient whose frustration was summarized in his testimony at a House of Representatives subcommittee [25]:

I am unable to secure any experimental drugs that may, in fact, prolong my life.

In addition to preceding the availability of reasonable evidence of efficacy, such requests precede the collection of safety data on a large number of patients. In such cases where even a preliminary estimate of the benefit/risk profile of the new drug is not available, treatment use of the investigational drug seems highly unwise due to the unknown benefits and unknown hazards of the drug. Dr. Young [1] summarized the conflict in such situations:

It is a fine line that public health officials must walk to protect the public from unsafe or useless drugs while allowing them access to some as yet unproven treatment that may be their last hope. The terrible disease AIDS has brought this issue to public scrutiny as never before.

Later in this same publication, Dr. Young [1] summarized the rationale for FDA's denial of treatment use:

Nevertheless, it would not be appropriate to make drugs widely available too early in the development process. While dying patients may be willing to 'try anything,' it would be irresponsible—and far from compassionate—to raise false hopes. The risks of a drug, as well as its benefits, must be measured very carefully. There are very few conditions, not even AIDS, that can't be made worse. . . It's not easy to be patient amid reports of dramatic results with a new drug for AIDS or Alzheimer's disease, for instance. But it's not always easy, or even possible, to tell whether those early findings are real.

VIII. SUMMARY

The final Treatment IND regulations which became effective in mid-1987 provided much needed rules regarding the treatment use of investigational new drugs. These regulations and the historical experience accumulated by FDA and corporate sponsors with treatment protocols have yielded a better understanding of the framework in which such use is appropriate. Equally important, treatment use of an investigational new drug provides an opportunity to explore a different aspect of the benefit/risk profile of the drug. Clearly, the desperately ill patients enrolled in a treatment protocol would have a different benefit/risk profile than those patients with predominantly non-serious or non-life-threatening disease who would be enrolled in conventional controlled clinical trials. Therefore, treatment use of an investigational new drug provides a means of expanding knowledge of the safety and efficacy of the drug through broadening of the target patient population in terms of severity and stage of disease. This promise of broader characterization of the properties of the drug, along with the humanitarian aspects of providing an investigational new drug to desperate patients, is the impetus for consideration of the proper place for treatment use protocols within the clinical drug development programs for each investigational new drug intended in part for the treatment of serious or life-threatening disease.

REFERENCES

1. Young FE. Experimental drugs for the desperately ill. *FDA Consumer*, p. 2, June 1987.
2. Young FE, Norris JA, Levitt JA, Nightingale SL. The FDA's new procedures for the use of investigational drugs in treatment. *JAMA 259*: 2267–2270 (1988).
3. Investigational New Drug, Antibiotic, and Biological Drug Product Regulations; Treatment Use and Sale; Final Rule. *Federal Register 52* (Number 99): 19466–19477 (May 22, 1987).
4. Nightingale SL. Final rule on treatment use and sale of investigational drugs. *JAMA 258*: 179 (1987).
5. Young FE, Nightingale SL. Information on Treatment INDs as they become available to the practitioner. *JAMA 260*: 247 (1988).
6. Young FE, Nightingale SL. FDA's newly designated Treatment INDs. *JAMA 260*: 224–225 (1988).
7. New Drug, Antibiotic, and Biologic, Drug Product Regulations; Final Rule. *Federal Register 52* (Number 53): 8798–8847 (March 19, 1987).
8. Treatment IND denials most often due to lack of safety & efficacy support, FDA's Temple tells AMA/FDA conference; Drug Division consultation suggested. *F-D-C Reports (The Pink Sheet)*, pages 6–7, February 22, 1988.
9. Investigational New Drug, Antibiotic, and Biological Drug Product Regulations; Subpart E—Procedures for Drugs Intended to Treat Life-Threatening and Severely Debilitating Illnesses. *Federal Register 53* (No. 204): 41516–41524 (October 21, 1988).
10. Johnstone JM. Treatment IND safety assessment: potential legal and regulatory problems. *Food Drug Cosmetic Law Journal 43*: 533–540 (1988).
11. Rodel PV. The compassionate use protocol as a research tool. *Controlled Clinical Trials 5*: 310 (1984).
12. Oraflex may have compassionate use, FDA Acting Com. Novitch tells Rep. Weiss. *F-D-C Reports (The Pink Sheet) 46* (Number 16): 12–13 (1984).
13. Newport isoprinosine studies have shown trend toward delay of "full blown AIDS". *F-D-C Reports (The Pink Sheet) 47* (Number 35): T&G-2 (1985).
14. Creagh-Kirk T, Doi P, Andrews E, Nusinoff-Lehrman S, Tilson H, Hoth D, Barry DW. Survival experience among patients with AIDS receiving zidovudine. Follow-up of patients in a compassionate plea program. *JAMA 260*: 3009–3015 (1988).
15. Beers DO. Emergency use INDs and IDEs: what is required? What are the risks? *Food Drug Cosmetic Law Journal 43*: 759–765 (1988).
16. Guidance for the Emergency Use of Unapproved Medical Devices; Availability. *Federal Register 50* (No. 204): 42866–42867 (October 22, 1985).
17. Appler WD. The FDA's Treatment IND rule—a glimpse into the future of drug regulation in the U.S.? *Food Drug Cosmetic Law Journal 43*: 649–658 (1988).
18. Treatment IND drug list should be made available. *F-D-C Reports (The Pink Sheet)*, T&G-2-3, February 22, 1988.

19. Expanded availability of investigational new drugs through a Parallel Track Mechanism for People with AIDS and HIV-Related Disease. Notice; Proposed policy statement. *Federal Register* 55 (Number 98): 20856–20860 (May 21, 1990).
20. Coverage of personal importations. Chapter 9–71. *Regulatory Procedures Manual.* TN 90-02 (December 11, 1989).
21. Obligations of Clinical Investigators of Regulated Articles. *Federal Register* 43 (Number 153): 35210–35236 (August 8, 1978).
22. Protection of Human Subjects; Informed Consent. *Federal Register 46* (Number 17): 8942–8980 (January 27, 1981) and 49 (Number 212): 43637–43638 (October 31, 1984).
23. Yarchoan R, Klecker RW, Weinhold KJ, Markham PD, Lyerly HK, Durack DT, Gelmann E, Lehrman SN, Blum RM, Barry DW, Shearer GM, Fischl MA, Mitsuya H, Bolognesi DP, Myers CE, Broder S. Administration of 3'-azido-3'-deoxythymidine, an inhibitor of HTLV-III/LAV replication, to patients with AIDS or AIDS-related complex. *Lancet 1*: 575–580 (1986).
24. FDA on isoprinosine in AIDS. *SCRIP World Pharmaceutical News*, Number 1001, p. 16 (May 22, 1985).
25. *U.S. News & World Report*, July 14, 1986, page 67.

part three

Issues in Managing
Clinical Drug Development

7

Maintenance of Continuity

> Future shock . . . the shattering stress and
> disorientation that we induce in individuals by
> subjecting them to too much change in too short time.
>
> *Alvin Toffler*

I. INTRODUCTION

Continuity is defined as (1) uninterrupted connection, succession, or union, and (2) persistence without essential change over time [1]. In drug development, continuity of the research program is that characteristic which enables completion of a research program with sufficient cohesiveness and integrity to supply valid answers to the questions posed in the objectives of the drug development plan. Achievement and maintenance of continuity in drug research is a challenge, particularly in the clinical component of drug development. The relatively long period of time from IND filing to NDA approval comprises a temporal basis for major challenges to continuity in clinical drug development.

Historically, the process of drug development has been segmentally organized in both the preclinical and clinical components. In such a segmental organization, a new chemical entity, or preferably a series of new chemical congeners, is evaluated for pharmacological activity. Compounds with acceptable selected activities undergo some preliminary toxicological and metabolic evaluation using various *in vitro* and *in vivo* systems. More extensive animal or *in vitro* pharmacology, toxicology, and drug metabolism evaluations may be performed concurrently with more than one leading candidate from a series of compounds. Despite the distinguishable and organizationally segmented activities performed by scientists from each basic research discipline, a new chemical entity often progresses through a multidisciplinary research team so that diverse activities can progress concurrently. Hence, development can occur as expeditiously as is feasible. These research teams generally strive to produce viable, sustained, high quality research within a given therapeutic area of drug development.

This preclinical research process identifies compounds for entry into clinical development. Ultimately, full clinical research programs will be conducted on appropriate compounds. As discussed in previous chapters, clinical drug development programs must generate a sufficiently large body of clinical data to establish an acceptable benefit/risk profile for the investigational drug.

Given this very brief overview of the sequence of activities in drug development, it is clear that multiple factors may contribute to a break in continuity of the drug development program. Problems in maintaining continuity arise due to turnover of personnel (e.g., medical monitors and investigators); evolving criteria for evaluation of disease processes about which pathophysiologic knowledge is rapidly increasing; and the sense that multicenter, Phase III clinical trials are monitored with less personal interest as they grow larger.

In order to establish some temporal context in which to solidify these notions on the importance of continuity, we reviewed information on the time course of drug development and regulatory document review. Table 1 lists the dates of NDA receipt by FDA and approval dates for a variety of new chemical entities approved since 1977. While this list is neither all inclusive nor necessarily a representative sample, it satisfies our goal of including a variety of compounds with which many practicing physicians, investigators, and industrial monitors will be familiar. These examples indicate that the FDA review time (i.e., the time from NDA receipt to approval) ranges from one to three and a half years. This observation is consistent with recent work by Spivey et al. [3] who reported the following median review times for NDAs on new chemical entities:

Year of Approval	Median Review Time (months)
1970	18
1971	19
1972	25
1973	21
1974	14

Year of Approval	Median Review Time (months)
1975	19
1976	22
1977	20
1978	18
1979	39
1980	20
1981	14
1982	10
1983	13

Further, our own experience with new chemical entities from each of these therapeutic classes listed in Table 1 is that the time from IND filing to NDA filing (i.e., the pre-NDA clinical trial period) ranges from approximately three to seven years). Taken together, these durations for the pre-NDA clinical trial period and the review period indicate that the sponsor and monitors can anticipate a five to ten year period from IND filing to approval of a safe and effective new chemical entity. This long period of time presents a substantial challenge to efforts to maintain continuity, particularly in view of the short average duration of employment (i.e., four to five years) of a monitor in a given position in the pharmaceutical industry. These numbers suggest that the average sponsor can anticipate turnover of up to two full monitoring staffs during the time from IND filing to NDA approval.

Clearly, there is a temporal basis for major challenges to continuity in clinical drug development. Moreover, it is unlikely that personnel turnover could be reduced sufficiently to enable individual personnel to bridge the discontinuities over time. Therefore, combatting discontinuity depends on understanding the intellectual basis for continuity in clinical research. Resolution of breaks in continuity of all etiologies depends upon the integrity of purpose of this intellect, which we will define as research mentality.

II. THE CONCEPT OF RESEARCH MENTALITY

Drug development is a scientific research process which originates with a new chemical entity and produces an ever-broadening, ever-deepening understanding of the new compound. In this regard, drug development is a science in that it shares the general property of all science, i.e., helping to satisfy man's desire to gain ever wider and deeper knowledge of the world around him [4]. Ideally, the drug development process progresses

Table 1. Summary of regulatory dates for a variety of new chemical entities.

Therapeutic Class	New Chemical Entity	NDA Number	NDA Receipt Date (mo-day-yr)	FDA Approval Date (mo-day-yr)
Cardiovascular	atenolol (Tenormin)	18240	12-21-78	08-19-81
	nifedipine (Procardia)	18482	04-30-80	12-31-81
	guanabenz (Wytensin)	18587	12-29-80	09-07-82
	captopril (Capoten)	18343	01-31-80	04-06-81
	labetalol (Trandate)	18686	08-24-82	08-01-84
	tocainide (Tonocard)	18257	12-19-79	11-09-84
	enalapril (Vasotec)	18998	09-16-83	12-24-85
Neuropharmacology	amoxapine (Asendin)	18021	04-14-77	09-22-80
	alprazolam (Xanax)	18276	03-02-79	10-16-81
	trazadone (Desyrel)	18207	10-11-78	12-24-81
	buprenorphine (Buprenex)	18401	11-01-79	12-29-81
	triazolam (Halcion)	17892		11-15-82

Anti-Infective	cefadroxil (Duracef)	50512	02-17-77	02-17-78
	ketoconazole (Nizoral)	18533	07-17-80	06-12-81
	acyclovir (Zovirax)	18604	06-09-81	03-29-82
	netilmicin (Netromycin)	50544	04-11-80	02-28-83
	ceftazidime (Fortaz)	50578	05-23-83	07-19-85
	butaconazole (Femstat)	19215	01-23-84	11-25-85
Gastrointestinal	cimetidine (Tagamet)	17920	07-16-76	08-16-77
	sucralfate (Carafate)	18333	07-02-79	10-30-81
	ranitidine (Zantac)	18703	03-10-82	06-09-83
Anesthesiology	atracurium (Tracrium)	18831	10-26-82	11-23-83
	sufentanil (Sufenta)	19050	06-17-83	05-04-84
	midazolam (Versed)	18654	12-15-82	12-20-85
Respiratory	bitolterol (Tornalate)	18770	07-20-82	12-28-84
	terfenadine (Seldane)	18949	03-01-83	05-08-85
Anti-Inflammatory	sulindac (Clinoril)	17911	06-30-76	09-27-78
	piroxicam (Feldene)	18147	03-31-78	04-06-82
	diflunisal (Dolobid)	18445	06-30-80	04-19-82

Source: Ref. 2.

until a complete package of information is constructed and everything is known about the drug. Unfortunately, real research processes are subject to limitations imposed by scarce resources of time, money, manpower, and intellectual energies. Therefore, the goal of the drug development process is to obtain an optimal package of information (i.e., all you can realistically know, given the constraints). Based on this optimal knowledge, the most rational use of a given drug can be developed.

We define the intellectual basis for continuity and generation of optimal knowledge as research mentality. With respect to clinical drug development, research mentality encompasses (1) an accumulative understanding of the available data from animal and human experiments, as well as the implications of these data; (2) a perspective on the optimal attainable knowledge about the drug; (3) a perspective on missing information or data that can not be collected (due to technological, ethical, or other barriers); (4) a sense of research priorities; and (5) temporal and conceptual understanding of both historical events and future plans. Thus, research mentality consists of the collective knowledge of available information and collective awareness of the potential of research in that field. Research mentality is the intellectual driving force of progressive research efforts.

We examine research mentality as the basis for continuity of research in drug development and the pursuit of optimal knowledge of a new drug. The characteristics of the predominant research mentality in both the basic research setting and the clinical research setting are compared. In addition, the four major classes of perturbations to research mentality, and hence continuity, are discussed.

III. RESEARCH MENTALITY AND DRUG DEVELOPMENT

A. Contrast in Research Mentalities of Basic Research versus Clinical Research

One of our fundamental assertions is that the clinical research process is more sensitive to perturbations and breaks in continuity than basic (i.e., preclinical) research. This contention is based on observations of the fundamental differences between the research mentality of clinical research and the research mentality of basic research. In basic research, there is a *collective* research mentality which is exercised, with respect to decision making, by a group of scientists comprising a *critical mass*. Critical mass is a primary characteristic of an effective preclinical research environment. Critical mass is defined as the minimum essential synergistic collection of collaborative, interdisciplinary personnel necessary to comprise a viable, intellectually vibrant, and sustained research mentality. In basic research, intellectual advances are achieved via a collective research mentality exercised by a critical mass. This notion has been emphasized in modern work on the nature of industrial America [5], as well as in work on pharmaceutical development [6]. An example of a pharmaceutical application of such critical masses is formation of the Sir James Black Foundation, a small group of approximately 20 scientists collaborating in discovery and development of novel therapies [7]. Their effort is receiving funding from Johnson and Johnson for 10 years.

A second characteristic of the preclinical research mentality is evident after reviewing the process through which many new hypotheses are generated. During times of advancing knowledge in basic research, decision making is non-algorithmic in nature. Kuhn [8] noted that advances in scientific research often seem to be a direct response to a crisis resulting from the overt failure of existing theories to solve a problem at hand. Similarly, he observed that new theories were rarely advanced in the absence of such crises. This process of scientific innovation in the face of crisis demonstrates another characteristic, i.e., the *initiative* nature of the basic research mentality. The basic research mentality uses the "research pentagon" for (1) reviewing existing information, (2) culling new information from this existing information, (3) collecting new data, (4) extrapolating new hypotheses and information from these three to experimentally untested situations, and (5) advancing new inductive hypotheses in response to unexplained data and crisis situations. Thus, the basic research mentality functions to innovate and expand knowledge, often in directions not anticipated by the application of deductive logic.

In contrast to the preclinical research mentality, the research mentality of clinical research is often substantially less collective than that of basic research. This critical difference in the operating intellect is partially fueled by the fact that decision making in the clinical setting generally does not depend on a critical mass of interdisciplinary experts. Clinical decision making is temporally sequential, algorithmic, and often individualistic in nature. Unlike the initiative nature of basic research, the mentality in the clinical setting is *responsive*. The clinical research mentality responds to the existing data in the decision-making algorithm, rather than constantly seeking to expand knowledge in the manner of the basic research mentality.

B. Need for a Collective Research Mentality in Clinical Research

The contrast between the basic research mentality and the clinical research mentality is clear. The clinical research mentality is *singular, temporally sequential, algorithmic, and responsive*. These characteristics generate a unidimensional mentality which can increase knowledge, but only in one dimension, i.e., a single linear dimension defined by the controlling intellectual constraints. The basic research mentality is *collective, temporally non-constrained, non-algorithmic, and initiative*. These characteristics generate a 3-dimensional mentality with enormous capacity to expand knowledge not only in the linear direction of existing knowledge, but also by expanding into the entire plane of existing knowledge and further expanding into other planes of knowledge in either a logical or, occasionally, illogical manner. This approach embraces the concepts of lateral thinking [9]. In order to develop optimal knowledge of a drug, drug developers must exploit expanding research mentality, initiative mentality, and critical mass much more extensively in the clinical research process. To do less is to fail to exploit the discoveries and innovations that continue to emerge on pathophysiologic and pharmacologic mechanisms.

Research mentality directs decision making in drug development. Moreover, research mentality must direct decision making at all levels of drug development if the pharmaceutical industry, like other evolving industries, is to utilize the creative intellects of personnel at all levels of the drug development process. The use of such creativity of all employees has been discussed in detail with respect to American industry by Kanter [5]. Since research mentality is responsible ideally for every level of decision made in an attempt to develop optimal knowledge of the drug, perturbations in the growth of the research mentality or deletions from the research mentality will affect the decision-making process and may displace the goal of developing optimal knowledge. Specific types of perturbations to the research mentality will be considered in the following section.

IV. PERTURBATIONS OF RESEARCH MENTALITY

As defined previously, research mentality is the intellectual basis of the approach toward assembling optimal knowledge about a drug. Potential perturbations of the research mentality can alter the degree of optimal knowledge which is achievable. Four classes of perturbations to research mentality have been identified. These classes are science-based, personnel-based, marketing-based, and regulation-based perturbations. Science-based perturbations consist of evolving knowledge in medical science. Personnel-based perturbations consist of personnel factors involving extracompany investigators, corporate research personnel, and corporate administrative personnel. Marketing-based perturbations consist of changes or deletions in research mentality primarily due to marketing considerations, rather than scientific considerations. Regulation-based perturbations consist of FDA-related factors. Table 2 lists some examples of reasons for perturbations in the research mentality from each of these four classes of perturbations. Each type of perturbation is discussed in more detail below.

A. Science-Based Perturbations

Since clinical drug development takes 4 to 10 years, there are numerous opportunities for both evolutionary and explosive change in science in the area of research. Our knowledge of the pathophysiology of disease processes, methods for diagnosis, methods for evaluation of the status of disease, and currently optimal therapy for some diseases are all medical science factors that change with time. Evolution of such medical knowledge occurs concurrently with development of a new drug and may comprise either a barrier or a boost to understanding the utility of the drug. For example, the American Psychiatric Association considered reclassification of the DSM-III diagnosis of generalized anxiety disorder in favor of incorporation in DSM-IV of more specific diagnoses [10]. Such a change could have either a profound effect or no effect on an ongoing anxiolytic drug development program, depending upon the basic diagnostic data collected and the degree to which this potential change was anticipated. As another example, it is reasonable to anticipate that advances in diagnostic imaging with PET (positron emission tomography), MRI (magnetic resonance imaging), SPECT, and other visualization technologies will further alter the diagnoses of psychiatric disorders by providing pathophysiologic evaluations of patients. Quantitative imaging and other technologies which enable cellular and molecular level characterization of pathophysiology will further alter medical science across diverse areas, including cardiology, gastroenterology, and neurology. Corporate research personnel must participate in the evolutionary and revolutionary process of science in order to maintain optimal preparedness for such perturbations.

B. Personnel-Based Perturbations

Changes in personnel can have a profound effect on research mentality. This effect occurs since loss of a scientist gives rise to a gap in the research mentality, unless there is someone else who understands and fully appreciates the same knowledge. As a result of personnel changes, the critical mass and, consequently, the research mentality are disrupted and diminished. In fact, the research mentality may diminish in excess of the quantity of expertise lost, especially if a viable critical mass is not sustained or reconstructed.

The segmental organization of drug discovery and development promotes a drug development process in which a new chemical entity is passed from chemistry to pharmacology to toxicology to clinical pharmacology to

Table 2. Reasons for breaks in continuity of a clinical research/drug development program.

A. General Issues:
  1. lack of explicit attention to continuity by investigators, monitors, sponsors, and FDA
  2. evolution of the data collection process (e.g., changes in case report forms as project progresses; data may be more detailed or less detailed as project progresses)
B. Scientific Factors:
  1. rapidly evolving knowledge of some disease processes
  2. rapidly evolving knowledge of methods to evaluate some disease processes
  3. controversy regarding methods to evaluate some diseases
  4. controversy regarding optimal therapy for some diseases
  5. development of an effective therapy so that a placebo-controlled trial may no longer be possible
  6. change in potential comparative drugs as recently approved drugs become available
C. Investigator Factors:
  1. deviation from protocol as his personal experience with the drug increases
  2. diminishing attention to intensity of observation and completion of case report forms as experience increases
  3. inadequate interest in uniformity of methods across multicenter trials
  4. diminishing vigilance to patient follow-up as experience increases
  5. inability to reproduce medical judgements (e.g., some patients with mild apparent hypersensitivity reactions may be discontinued, but others are continued)
  6. changes with time as project progresses (tendency toward increased investigator complacency; less attention to detail; increased tendency to assume that the drug is safe and effective)
  7. program gets larger, involves more investigators, and becomes less personal
D. Monitor Factors:
  1. minimal interest and knowledge of the global project objectives of clinical research
  2. inadequate attention to detail due to reliance on data quality control and quality assurance procedures to detect errors
  3. inadequate attention to capturing the basis for a change in project direction
  4. competition among monitors to the exclusion of information sharing
  5. inadequate reward for key monitors
  6. lack of documentation for many, apparently minor decisions (e.g., selection of certain indications, exclusion of selected patients, factors for stratification or lack of stratification of patients on admission to a study)

Table 2. (*Continued*)

7. changes in personnel (e.g., promotion of a monitor to a more senior position with another project)
8. monitor-to-monitor variations in style, aggressiveness, and compulsiveness
9. changes with time as project progresses (tendency toward increased monitor complacency; less attention to detail; increased tendency to assume that the drug is safe and effective)
10. program gets larger, involves more investigators and more monitors, and becomes less personal
E. Sponsor Factors:
1. lack of formalized project teams to assemble a critical mass, define project team member responsibilities, and prioritize multiple project tasks
2. hierarchical structure that excludes some clinical monitors from project team meetings
3. failure to reward key monitors, project team members, and investigators
4. inadequate funding allocated to investigator meetings and publication activities
5. licensure of a drug to another sponsor for development
6. subcontracting of a drug to a contract company for development
F. FDA Factors:
1. evolving criteria for drug review
2. changing standards of practice (IND/NDA Rewrites)
3. change in the specific medical officer responsible for review

clinical development to post-marketing surveillance. While this organizational structure succeeds in recognizing the specialized nature of each task, it can promote unidirectional flow of information and hence comprise a substantial barrier to formation of a contiguous interdisciplinary critical mass and research mentality.

Major personnel-based perturbations of the research mentality can occur after achievement of a milepost in the drug development process. Such mileposts include filing an IND, end-of-Phase II conference, pre-NDA conference, NDA filing, and NDA approvability. Achievement of a milepost may be followed by changes in some personnel. For example, there may be addition of staff after a promising end-of-Phase II conference. Since these new staff members have no experience with this drug and perhaps no experience in this therapeutic area, their presence will perturb, at least initially, the continuity of the development process. As another example, NDA approval is such a major milepost that some research administrators believe the drug development process is essentially complete.

Indeed, the process is complete in terms of being able to supply drug to a larger patient population. However, contributions from personnel who have developed the research mentality are still needed to assure a smooth transition into post-marketing studies and proper planning for potential line extensions. The time of NDA approval is a time for major breeches in continuity due to personnel changes and hence great breeches in the research mentality. In the interest of applying the most experienced scientists to other critical projects, scientists who have directed projects through an NDA are often re-assigned to other projects soon after drug approval. Further, several companies have organizational structures that separate the monitors and investigators conducting the post-marketing research program from the personnel who conducted the pre-NDA program. Such structures promote a fragmented research mentality and breaks in continuity.

Optimal knowledge about a drug has not yet been attained at the time of approval of the NDA. Ideally, approval of the NDA coincides with the time of collection of a database which comprises substantial evidence that the drug has an acceptable benefit/risk profile. Traditionally, approval of a NDA is a rather well-defined process compared with the goals of a post-marketing research program. Post-marketing research consists of the difference between optimal knowledge and the knowledge contained in the acceptable benefit/risk profile which enabled approval of the drug. Decisions made in the post-marketing period may further generate personnel-based breaks in continuity. Indeed, the research team which may have assembled the basis for drug approval may be dismantled following approval. This is an extreme example of a continuity problem.

C. Marketing-Based Perturbations

Decisions to redirect the research effort, based principally on marketing considerations, may eliminate or ignore a portion of the research mentality that was developed to provide the current understanding of the drug. This situation gives rise to marketing-based perturbations of the research mentality which can derail the process of developing an optimal understanding of a given drug.

The business applications of clinical research must be as independent as possible of the research mentality. Too often, business decisions are made despite the consequent implicit necessity to drop a portion of the research mentality. Such decisions may be made to accomplish a short-term goal which may not be compatible with attainment of optimal knowledge as the long-term goal. For example, Reidenberg [11] suggested that it is misleading to rely on projections from market research as a means to prioritize development programs for novel drugs. In order to reconcile such conflicts, business decisions must be factored into the research mentality, but not control the decision-making process in the research mentality. Research mentality must remain intellectually ahead of business concerns in order to avoid domination by business concerns. The research mentality at some point needs to become business sensitive so that it can help to optimize sales, but it should never be business directed. Clearly, a portion of the research mentality can be prioritized in light of business factors in order to take account of the realities of business pressures.

It is noteworthy that exclusive attention of the research mentality to marketing considerations will rarely expand the research mentality. Marketing considerations usually require information about things that are already known or deducible from the existing knowledge base, despite the fact that this information may not be widely disseminated.

D. Regulation-Based Perturbations

Drug approval is a regulatory process conducted under the auspices of the FDA. Evolving criteria for drug safety and efficacy and changing standards of practice (e.g., the NDA rewrites [12]) are sources of regulatory perturbations to the research mentality.

The Food, Drug, and Cosmetic Act of 1938 and the subsequent amendments to this act commission the Secretary of Health and Human Services and hence the Food and Drug Administration to perform one of the least enviable and most complex regulatory tasks the government can undertake. Among the FDA's tasks is the responsibility for assuring the provision of substantial evidence of safety and efficacy for all prescription and over-the-counter pharmaceuticals.

> Sec. 505 [355]. (a) No person shall introduce or deliver for introduction into interstate commerce any new drug, unless an approval of an application filed pursuant to subsection (b) is effective with respect to such drug. (b) Any person may file with the Secretary an application with respect to any drug subject to the provisions of subsection (a). Such persons shall submit to the Secretary as a part of the application (1) full reports of the investigations which have been made to show whether or not such drug is safe for use and whether such drug is effective for use; [13]

The complexity and difficulty of this particular task arises from the multidisciplinary nature of the medical sciences in general and pharmaceutical development in particular. Scientific advances in many areas interact to improve our understanding of pathophysiology, diagnosis, and pharmacotherapy. As medical science advances, the FDA must utilize these new understandings in the process of evaluating the safety and efficacy of new drugs. Although the FDA usually makes a diligent attempt to communicate the regulatory requirements for new drugs through the Code of Federal Regulations, guidelines, and meetings with representatives of industrial sponsors, the FDA must utilize the most viable and current understanding that medical science can provide at the time they are evaluating a new drug for approval. The FDA keeps the medical community apprised of the regulatory changes it proposes and subsequently adopts. Despite such communication, these changes constitute regulation-based perturbations to the research mentality. In this regard, the so-called NDA rewrites imposed several major changes in the regulatory considerations governing drug development. For example, these new regulations increase the scope of reporting of adverse events during the NDA review period. These new requirements change the drug development process. Additional personnel must be allocated to this function and personnel will require additional training to accomplish these new requirements. Also, additional personnel are likely to be required in several other areas (e.g., clinical data processing) to meet these new standards. Few can legitimately argue that these new regulations are unreasonable or ill-advised. Implementation of such regulations mean that development of a new drug will require increased resources to accomodate these regulatory changes.

While the NDA rewrites represent a major perturbation to drug development, more subtle changes in FDA's positions also constitute perturbations to the research mentality surrounding a given drug. These more subtle regulatory perturbations are often the result of an evolving knowledge in a given research area. For example, the issue of ulcer recurrence during long-term therapy of duodenal ulcer disease has received considerable attention recently [14-17]. At one point, one study design had been used in all of the long-term therapy trials in patients with duodenal ulcer disease. This design was endorsed at one point by the FDA. As a result of a changing understanding of the disease and its therapies, this design has come under considerable scrutiny. The position of the FDA and some investigators on this study design has changed. This change will have significant impact on continuing efforts to evaluate long-term therapy in patients with this disease. Similar changes may occur in a variety of other specific therapeutic areas. In fact, some of these changes are the result of research sponsored by the pharmaceutical industry. Since such changes result from a new understanding in a given disease area, pharmaceutical companies may be left with little choice but to accept the rationale for these changes and incorporate this information into their research mentalities.

V. MEASURES TO PREVENT AND COUNTERACT BREECHES IN RESEARCH MENTALITY

Having identified four classes of potential perturbations to research mentality and continuity, some approaches can be used to minimize the impact of perturbations on the research mentality. Research mentality must be maintained and it must continue to expand if it is to provide an ongoing basis for decision-making on the discovery, development, and use of new therapies. In most cases, research mentality will evolve in a manner consistent with its focus on the achievement of optimal knowledge about the drug. In this context of evolving research mentality, we must return to the critical mass concept.

Critical mass was defined previously as the minimum essential synergistic collection of collaborative, interdisciplinary personnel necessary to comprise a viable, sustained, dynamic research mentality. Changes in personnel comprising the critical mass must not alter the viability of the collective research mentality. One purpose of the critical mass is to detect when they are, in fact, challenged with a potential perturbation. The critical mass can then actively decide whether or not to change research priorities in full recognition of the fact that their goal remains to achieve optimal knowledge. In this way, changes imposed on the development of the research mentality are made consciously and with prospective thought regarding the potential impact of this change on attainment of optimal knowledge. Such a change may require that information previously collected be re-evaluated. In the event that errors occur in decision making, the critical mass can trace the basis for such decisions and redirect the research process.

The potential for discontinuity arises when the research mentality evolves either by inertia alone or by inertia with input from a non-critical mass. In such cases, the connection between research mentality and the goal of optimal knowledge has been breeched. Such breeches can be minimized in a number of ways. For each source of perturbation described previously, Table 3 summarizes some preventative and counteractive measures useful in maintaining continuity. Many of these measures are relatively obvious and do not warrant discussion. However, some discussion is warranted regarding the project team system as a mechanism for assembling critical mass. More extensive information on project team systems is provided in another chapter.

A. Project Teams

Within the last ten years, there has been some recognition of limitations of the "person mentality" as opposed to a collective research mentality

Table 3. Counteractive measures to facilitate maintenance of continuity.

A. General Issues:
   1. investigator, monitor, sponsor, and FDA awareness of the need for continuity
B. Scientific Factors:
   1. evaluate changes or evolving patterns of medical practice for impact on long-term research programs
   2. collect sufficient raw data (medical history, physical examination, mental status examination, laboratory tests, etc.) to enable reconstruction of the presenting patient
C. Investigator Factors:
   1. meetings of all monitors to coordinate investigator selection and topics for discussion at prestudy visits
   2. meetings of investigators for multicenter trials
   3. frequent, periodic updates of Investigators Brochure to disseminate information to investigators
   4. maintenance of a database on investigators performance
   5. identification of key project investigators with efforts to reward their continued presence in their roles
D. Monitor Factors:
   1. several people must know the details of a project (e.g., use non-doctoral personnel as assistants to senior personnel)
   2. multiple monitor sign-off on completed case report forms and data checking in order to promote maintenance of vigilance
   3. use prototype reports for data analysis
   4. maintain current, detailed Clinical Development Plan via periodic updates to capture the rationale of the developing project and project directional changes
   5. allow orientation phase for new monitoring personnel
   6. maintain project diary with dates and descriptions of project-guiding decisions
   7. periodic monitor meetings to share monitoring practices in order to achieve uniform vigilance
   8. periodic research discussion groups and publication efforts to maintain high monitor interest
   9. documentation of precedent-setting monitoring decisions with description of the logical base for the decisions
   10. identification of key project monitors with efforts to reward their continued presence in their roles
E. Sponsor Factors:
   1. use a project team approach to assemble a critical mass
   2. include monitors in project team meetings in order to encourage maintenance of personal interest
   3. identification of key project monitors and investigators with efforts to reward their continued presence in their roles

Table 3. (*Continued*)

4. allocate sufficient funding for monitor meetings, multicenter investigator meetings, and research discussion/publication activities
5. develop drugs under subcontract or co-licensure agreements only if intense collaboration of personnel comprising the critical masses of both parties can be achieved

F. FDA Factors:
   1. periodic meetings for presentation of data and updated Project Plans
   2. periodic conference calls for information exchange on relevant specific issues
   3. attend Advisory Committee hearings in order to monitor changing FDA personnel, philosophies, and standards

maintained by a critical mass. In view of the advantages of a critical mass, many pharmaceutical companies have adopted a project team system. For example, a project team may consist of basic research, medical, regulatory, biostatistical, marketing, and administrative personnel whose time is in part committed to a specific project, i.e., clinical development of a particular drug. There are several reasons for the increasing importance of the project team system in the pharmaceutical industry (Table 4).

The project team system can render clinical research less perturbable since there are more people informed about a greater breadth of the project. To withstand potential perturbations, the key to a project team system

Table 4. Reasons for increasing importance of the project team system in the pharmaceutical industry.

1. longer and costlier drug development cycles
2. increasing complexity of modern science necessitates a large critical mass of experts and skills
3. emphasis on near-term productivity rather than longer-term exploratory research
4. increasing external forces (regulatory requirements and consumer group pressures
5. growing impact of licensing and technology transfer groups
6. concern for orphan drugs and orphan indications
7. need for increased efficiency of R&D's productivity
8. shift of certain research to outside the U.S. with consequent need for coordinated international drug development
9. need for R&D management to maintain a motivated and creative staff

Source: Modified after Ref. 18.

is to instill the notion that the members are not charged with completing some specific task with this compound, but rather they are charged with maintaining the research mentality on this compound and the connection between the research mentality and attaining optimal knowledge about this compound. Their most important function is to detect potential deviations in the evolution of the research mentality and judge whether these deviations are beneficial to attainment of optimal knowledge. To this end, effective project teams require redundancy in order to avoid losses in critical mass and research mentality.

The project team is a multifaceted unit. If the team is responsible for maintaining the research mentality, it must accept the multidisciplinary nature of research efforts. The project team itself must become a critical mass and, more importantly, must spawn, nurture, and incorporate separate critical research masses in the required activities (e.g., basic research, clinical research, and regulatory affairs). If the project team incorporates the critical masses responsible for these various activities, then it will be possible for the team to withstand some personnel changes without sacrificing the evolution of the research mentality. If assembled and commissioned as described, project teams can mitigate most challenges to the research process except for administrative dissolution of the research team.

B.   Breaks in Research Mentality at the Time of Approval

The clinical research process does not end when the drug is approved. The approval point represents a point in time when a subset of information defining an acceptable benefit/risk profile has been assembled. Subsequent post-marketing research consists of the difference between optimal knowledge about the drug and the information contained in the acceptable benefit/risk profile. The mission, post-approval, is for the critical mass to maintain continuity by evaluating the information contained within that gap, prioritizing, and redirecting the research efforts. In the absence of such actions, the research mentality on a compound may be abandoned post-approval and continuity of post-marketing research may not be achievable. Such breaks in continuity are identifiable when the ongoing clinical research program fails to develop new information about the drug or replicates the same research programs that either failed or succeeded previously.

VI.   SUMMARY

We have discussed the importance of continuity in the clinical drug development process. Continuity acquires increasing importance in today's resource-limited research environment. There are clear limitations of time, money, and manpower which necessitate that we exploit the broadest possible intellect in order to optimize utility of the research and the drug. We have termed this intellect the research mentality and we have described the purpose of the drug development process as collection of an optimal package of information on the drug. We contend that if the research mentality is properly developed and properly nurtured, it will provide not only the information to direct the ongoing, evolving decision-making process in drug research, but also accumulate an aggregate knowledge both to optimize utility of a given drug and to provide marketing with the information to apprise their audience about that utility.

Unfortunately, there are many challenges to maintaining continuity. We have enumerated a few of these likely perturbations and we have listed some solutions to some of these perturbations. Clearly, the ongoing evolution of science and medicine must be integrated into the research mentality and thereby into the drug development process if knowledge about a given drug is to be useful to physicians. Science-based challenges to continuity continue throughout the life of a given drug. In fact, it can be argued that the useful life of a given drug is in serious jeopardy when continued expansion of our knowledge base on that drug is stopped either implicitly or explicitly. Clearly, one means to mitigate scientific perturbations is to foster participation of research personnel in their scientific and medical fields of expertise. In this way, the evolving research mentality concerning a specific drug acquires an anticipatory nature; changes in the research community will be factored into the sponsor's decision-making process to expand the research mentality before those changes are actually implemented in the practice of medicine.

It is difficult to be anticipatory of regulation-based challenges to continuity. Changes in the regulations are intended to improve the quality of information available to the FDA and prescribing physicians. These changes often occur in response to new scientific understanding concerning particular diseases or drug categories. Thus, the most widely available mechanisms to control the impact of any regulation-based perturbations are (1) to encourage research personnel to maintain a participatory role in the scientific community and (2) to promote information exchange concerning any changes in FDA's guidelines or policies. Such actions will help to assure that contingency plans are made to accomodate potential regulatory changes. Changes in the positions of regulatory agencies are often clearly justified and, in such cases, are usually implemented long before formal guidelines or regulations are issued. Thus, prior agreement based on an outmoded understanding of the required information is, realistically, of little value.

Marketing-based perturbations of continuity are a common problem and, in some respects, the least acceptable. Marketing-based perturbations are in sharp contrast to marketing-influenced research which exploits the research mentality, but does not divert the research mentality from its goal of an optimal understanding concerning a given drug. Market-support clinical trials generally attempt to exploit and further highlight a portion or subset of the information contained in the research mentality. Such research can be resource intensive for short periods of time (in general, less than two years) even for drugs such as antihypertensives which require relatively long-term studies for individual patients (e.g., four months to one year in a given study). If these types of studies become the predominant consumer of resources available for continued clinical drug development, the research mentality may fail to expand towards its optimal package of information. Under these circumstances, marketing-directed research constitutes a perturbation of the research mentality.

Obviously, control of such marketing-based perturbations is very difficult in a profit-motivated industry. Providing research to support marketing of a product is clearly in the financial interest of the company. Also, it is in the best interest of marketing to have an optimal package of information. However, optimal information is a long-term goal. Thus, the temptation to divert resources to market support is high and the short-term rewards seem great, but the long-term adverse impact on the research mentality for a particular drug may be irreparable. Of course, marketing will not perturb the research process if the critical mass project team provides the information that marketing can exploit.

Maintaining an awareness of the potential for marketing-based perturbations can mitigate their impact. However, a more durable solution is to promote participation of research personnel in their scientific and medical disciplines and to promote their interaction with the marketing personnel responsible for development of the marketing profile of a given drug. Again, by fostering the involvement of research personnel in the overall scientific community and marketing interactions, the drug development program will anticipate the needs of marketing, thereby enabling provision of sufficient information to develop an effective marketing program. While some marketing-directed research will always be conducted in this profit-motivated industry, it may be possible for such research efforts to be somewhat anticipatory and therefore contribute to the expansion of the research mentality. Such efforts would not consume the dominant portion of the resources available to research.

The personnel responsible for shaping the research mentality are the most important means of protecting against continuity problems. Consequently, personnel-based perturbations to the research mentality have far-ranging impact. Many companies attempt to achieve stability of personnel. However, personnel-related issues can not be limited to a consideration of programs developed to promote longevity of employment. In fact, many of the attempts to maintain an individual in a company will require administrative shifts that will be advantageous to the individual's career growth, while clearly perturbing the research mentality. Thus, it is important to establish a research process which is relatively insensitive to personnel changes. In this regard, establishing a collective intellect with a critical mass of personnel from different scientific disciplines should provide a viable research mentality, maximum opportunity to expand knowledge of the drug, and minimum risk of the previously identified perturbations. The opportunity for challenges from any the four major perturbations is most critically influenced by lack of a critical mass.

The project team concept provides a management tool with the potential to facilitate formation of a critical mass for a specific drug. Each of the component parts of the project team must be a self-perpetuating critical mass. Thus, the project team must conceptually be expanded to include all members of the research staff who are contributing to the research mentality. This structure requires a conscious effort to have some overlapping individual responsibilities in order to assure a certain minimum level of redundancy within each discipline.

In contemporary basic and clinical research settings, formation of a critical mass to develop a collective research mentality is the predominant approach to drug development. While one renowned individual may form the cornerstone around which a research program is developed, it seems increasingly rare for significant research to be performed in isolation. Thus, it can be argued that failure to develop a critical mass in any portion of the drug development process greatly jeopardizes the attainable level of success. Promoting continued scientific development of personnel contributing to the research mentality and charging the critical mass with maintenance of this research mentality appear to be the means by which the drug development process can avoid fatal disruptions of continuity.

REFERENCES

1. *Webster's Ninth New Collegiate Dictionary.* Springfield, MA: Merriam-Webster Inc., 1984.
2. Product Information Coordination Staff, Office of Management, Center for Drugs and Biologics, Food and Drug Administration. *New Drug Evaluation Statistical Report.* Springfield, VA: National Technical Information Service of the U.S. Department of Commerce. October, 1985 and March, 1986.

3. Spivey RN, Lasagna L, Trimble AG. New drug applications: how long to gain approval. *Clin. Pharmacol. Ther. 37*: 361–366 (1985).
4. Hempel CG. *Philosophy of Natural Science*. Englewood Cliffs, NJ: Prentice-Hall, Inc., 1966, page 2.
5. Kanter RM. *The Change Masters*. New York: Simon and Schuster, 1983.
6. Bartholini G. Organization of industrial drug research. In: *Decision Making in Drug Research* (Gross F, ed.). New York: Raven Press, pp. 123–146 (1983).
7. A visit to Sir James Black—the Schwartz commentary. *Scrip* (No. 1531), pp. 15–16 (July 13, 1990).
8. Kuhn TS. *The Structure of Scientific Revolutions*. Chicago: University of Chicago Press, p. 75 (1970).
9. de Bono E. *Lateral Thinking: Creativity Step by Step*. New York: Harper & Row, Publishers, 1970.
10. Spitzer R. DSM-IV. Presented at: 139th annual meeting of the American Psychiatric Association. Washington, DC. May, 1986.
11. Reidenberg MM. The state of drug development in the United States in 1990: a view from the academic community. *Clin. Pharmacol. Ther. 48*: 1–9 (1990).
12. New Drug and Antibiotic Regulations. *Federal Register 50* (Number 36): 7452–7519 (February 22, 1985).
13. *Federal Food, Drug and Cosmetic Act*. Washington, D.C.: U.S. Government Printing Office, 1979.
14. Elashoff JD, Koch GG, Chi GYH. Designing a clinical trial to demonstrate prevention of ulcer recurrence or other partially unobservable outcomes. Presented at: International Biometrics Meeting. August, 1986.
15. Elashoff JD, Koch GG, Chi GYH. Designing a clinical trial to demonstrate prevention of ulcer recurrence: modelling simulation approaches. *Statistics in Medicine 7*: 877–888 (1988).
16. Day SJ. Optimal placebo response rates for comparing two binomial proportion. *Statistics in Medicine 7*: 1187–1194 (1988).
17. Whitehead J. The analysis of relapse clinical trials, with application to a comparison of two ulcer treatments. *Statistics in Medicine 8*: 1439–1454 (1989).
18. Faust RE. Research planning and development perspectives. In: *The Clinical Research Process in the Pharmaceutical Industry* (Matoren GM, ed.). New York: Marcel Dekker Inc., Chapter 2, pp. 33–50, 1984.

8

Project Management Systems to Establish Continuity and Critical Mass

> Science bestowed immense new powers on man,
> and, at the same time, created conditions
> which were largely beyond his comprehension and
> still more beyond his control.
>
> *Sir Winston Churchill*

I. INTRODUCTION

The multidisciplinary nature of clinical drug development and the many years needed for development are two major factors that render the clinical drug development process susceptible to breaks in continuity and challenges of interdisciplinary coordination. Breaks in continuity have impact on drug development programs ranging from temporary disruptions of minor inconvenience to rendering a clinical trial program useless as support for approval of the drug. In an effort to minimize discontinuities and facilitate interdisciplinary coordination, various project management systems have been implemented in the pharmaceutical industry. Three such systems are the scientist-intensive, resource management, and critical mass systems. The basic characteristics of each system are summarized in this chapter. The unique deficiencies of the scientist-intensive and resource management approaches are presented. Optimization of a project and continuity in clinical drug development can be achieved by a multidisciplinary project team having critical mass. Critical mass project teams are the best means to attain both the short-term goal of evaluating the safety and efficacy of a compound (to provide the benefit/risk assessment necessary for drug approval) and the long-term goal of research equity.

Although previous chapters have presented information on the overall drug development process, a brief review of the history of drug development will provide an understanding of the motivation for using critical mass-based approaches to drug development.

II. HISTORICAL PERSPECTIVE ON DRUG DEVELOPMENT

Any perspective on the drug development process must recognize the young age of this process. The necessity to prove safety of drugs prior to marketing was not mandated until 1938 with the passage of the Federal Food Drug and Cosmetic Act. The necessity to prove efficacy was mandated for most drug classes less than 30 years ago with the Kefauver-Harris amendments of 1962. The drug development process continues to undergo evolution as indicated most obviously by the so-called proposed good clinical practice regulations [1-3], the NDA rewrites implemented in 1985 [4], and the IND rewrites of 1987 [5].

In the face of this relative youth, the pharmaceutical industry has developed rapidly. Administratively, the research component of the industry is often segmentally organized. This administrative organization produces a segmental drug development process (Figure 1) that is susceptible to breaks in continuity as compounds are passed from one segment of the research organization to another. Drug synthesis ordinarily occurs in a medicinal chemistry section, although chemical leads may come from other sources within a pharmaceutical company, as well as outside the company. The new chemical entity or a congeneric series of new chemical entities will undergo preliminary evaluation in pharmacology and toxicology. Those compounds with desirable activities will also be evaluated in the drug metabolism unit. Through evaluations in pharmacology and drug metabolism, the chemical structure/activity relationships will evolve and ultimately a series of compounds will be produced with varying degrees of the desired profile of activity. More detailed pharmacologic evaluation and drug metabolism studies, as well as expanded toxicological testing in higher species, will be used to select candidates that should progress for more extensive toxicological evaluation and be considered for clinical development.

One or more candidates from a series may be selected for human pharmacologic evaluation. The lead compound would be filed for an investigational new drug application (i.e., IND). Early human pharmacology trials would assess both the desirable and undesirable pharmacologic activities of the compound. Based on the human pharmacology and animal toxicology data, a decision can be made to progress one or more of the candidates into further Phase I/II testing. The purpose of clinical phar-

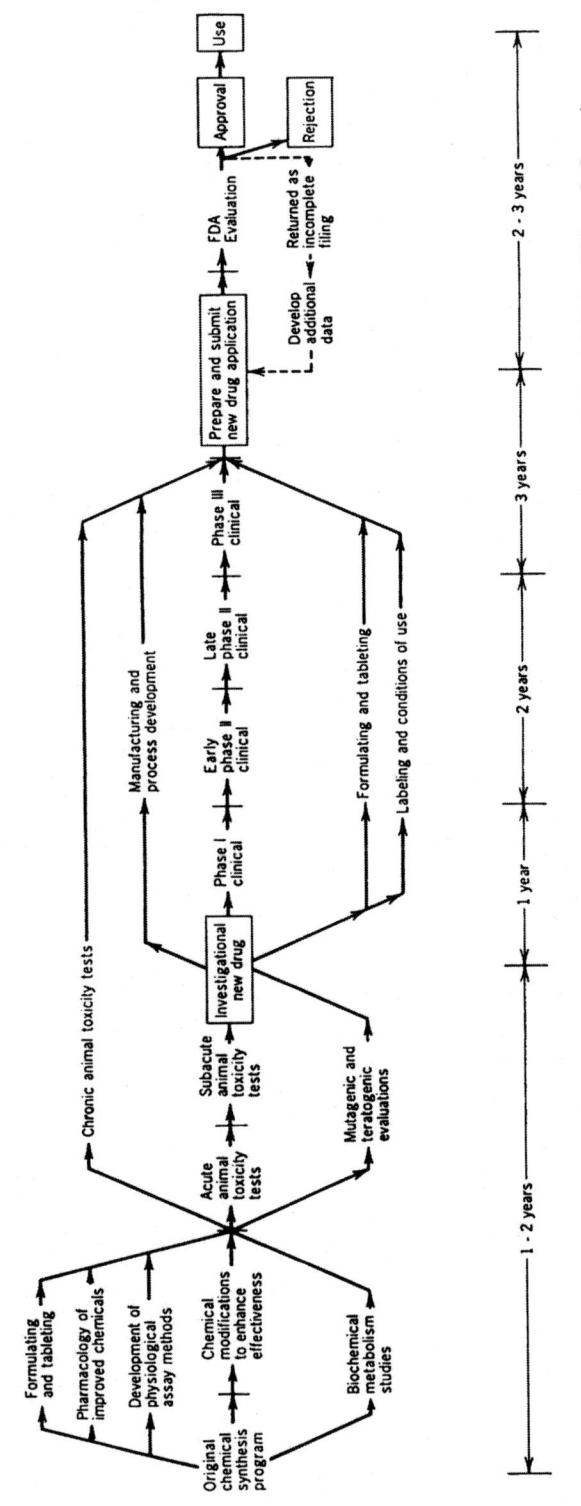

Figure 1. Illustration of the sequential drug development process in the U.S. (From Ref. 23, with permission of John Wiley & Sons.)

macological testing is to define the pharmacologic and toxicologic properties of a new chemical entity in humans and to assess the magnitude of separation between the therapeutic dose-response and toxic dose-response curves for each new chemical entity [6]. Generally, the compound with the most favorable profile will be fully characterized with respect to its therapeutic dose-response properties.

Ultimately, a decision will be reached, based on benefit/risk considerations, on whether the compound should continue through development toward a new drug application. Clinical development would then progress utilizing the dose range provided from earlier clinical studies. Placebo-controlled trials or active-controlled trials would be conducted in patients with the target disease in order to define the benefit/risk profile of the new chemical entity in the target population. A new drug application would be assembled based on data available from preclinical and clinical research. When it becomes apparent that a compound is likely to progress to an approvable new drug application, a post-marketing research plan should be developed and implemented in late Phase III with continuation into the post-marketing period.

The drug development process described above is sequential in that the drug progresses sequentially from chemistry to pharmacology to toxicology to human pharmacology to clinical development to post-marketing research.

III. THREE TYPES OF PROJECT MANAGEMENT

The sequential nature of the drug development process, hierarchical organizational structure of the pharmaceutical industry, and multidisciplinary nature of pharmaceutical development foster considerable challenges for coordination among scientists representing various contributory disciplines. In an effort to mitigate this coordination problem, pharmaceutical companies have implemented various project team approaches. A project team consists of a collection of individuals from different disciplines who have been assigned to work in a collegial manner to foster progress on their project. Comparisons can be made among three principal project team approaches to clinical drug development: scientist-intensive (Figure 2), resource management (Figure 3), and critical-mass based (Figure 4). Some of the principal characteristics of these three approaches are listed in Table 1.

The segmental nature of the drug development process has historically reinforced a *scientist-intensive* clinical drug development scheme (Figure 2). This approach establishes a medical scientist as the pivotal operative who receives information from other scientific departments. The scientist-

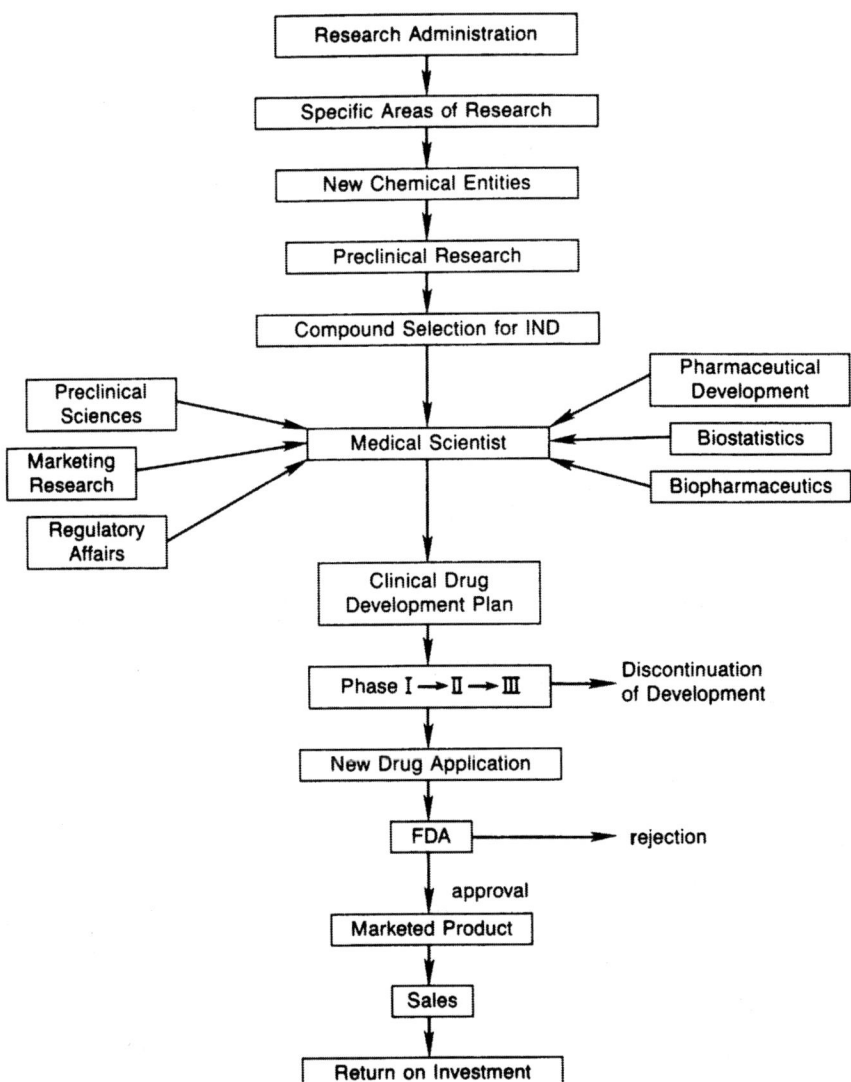

Figure 2. Schematic diagram of individual scientist-intensive clinical drug development system.

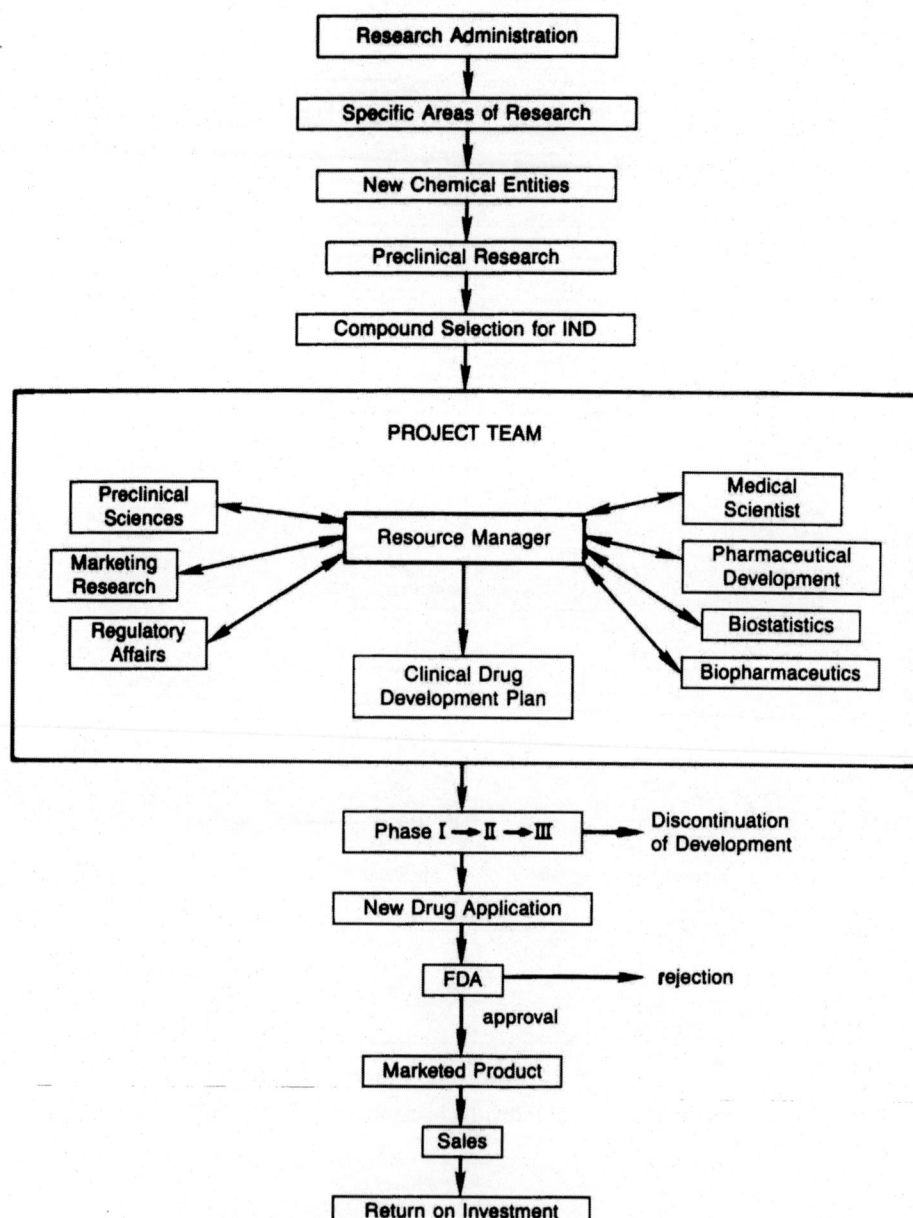

Figure 3. Schematic diagram of resource manager type of clinical drug development system.

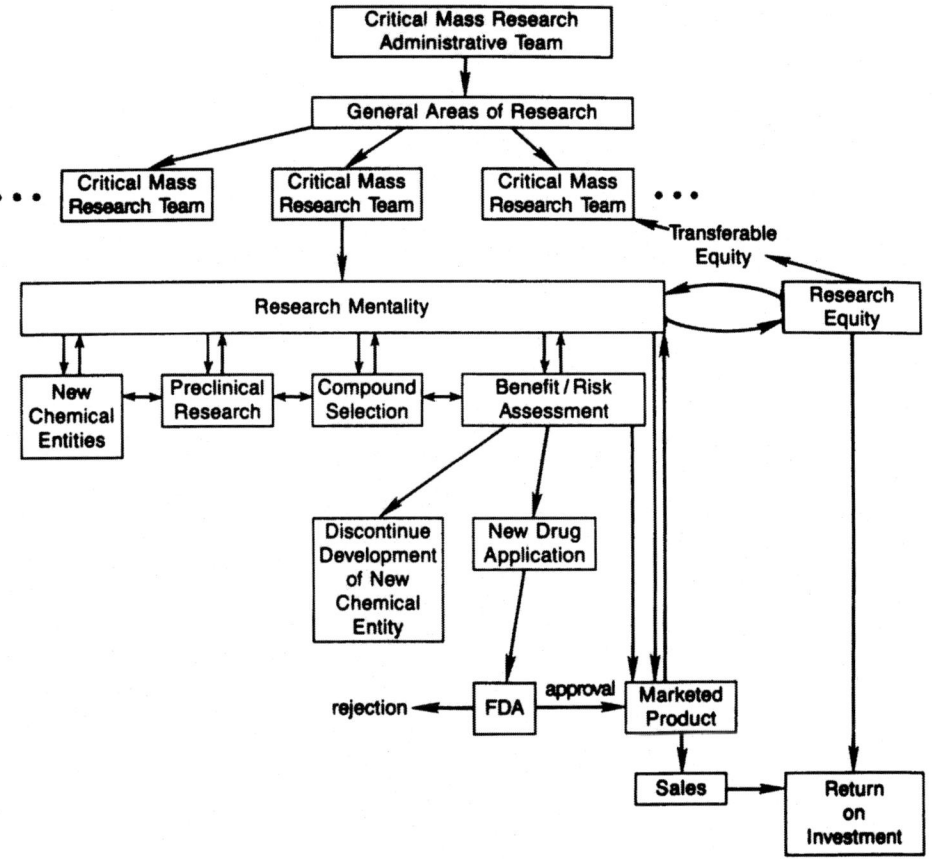

Figure 4. Schematic diagram of critical mass-based clinical drug development system.

intensive approach retains the sequential feature of drug development and uses primarily unidirectional communication. The approach can be highly perturbable, especially by loss or reassignment of the medical scientist.

The *resource management* system places increased emphasis on the interactive, interdisciplinary nature of drug development (Figure 3). It establishes a resource manager as the pivotal operative within a project team. Such a system functions principally to coordinate implementation and conduct of the drug development plan with the goal of making the drug development process cost-effective and expedient in developing approvable drugs. The resource manager may or may not be trained principally as a scientist. The scientific strength and integrity of purpose of

Table 1. Characteristics of three project team approaches to clinical drug development.

Project Team Approach	Characteristics
Scientist-intensive	1. medical scientist is the pivotal operative in clinical drug development 2. non-medical members of project have service functions 3. personnel are committed entirely to that project 4. highly perturbable to discontinuities by loss of medical scientist and limited communication due to segmental structure
Resource-management	1. resource manager is the pivotal operative in clinical drug development 2. project team members provide expertise in their respective fields; integration function is done by resource manager 3. resource managers across all development programs resolve resource conflicts 4. perturbable due to limited communication among scientists from different fields 5. limited redundancy of knowledge base
Critical-mass based	1. the research team is the pivotal operative in clinical drug development 2. collective information is available to all team members 3. minimal perturbability of critical mass is maintained due to redundancy of knowledge base 4. clinical studies directed toward benefit/risk assessment 5. system generates research mentality and research equity 6. research mentality and research equity can be applied by research administration to other areas of research without a negative impact on the source project

work contributed to the project from each specific discipline are judged solely by the respective contributor himself since he is the project team's designated authority in that discipline. The resource manager establishes bidirectional informational exchange with individual scientists on the project team. However, direct interactions among team scientists are not critical to conduct of the project. Therefore, like the scientist-intensive approach, the resource management system is highly dependent on an individual person. Resource managers for different projects communicate in order to minimize and resolve conflicts for shared resources. The resource managers are responsible for apprising research administration of project status, resource requirements, and delays or conflicts within a given project or imposed by other projects. Such a project team is very similar to the project teams implemented in traditional sequential enterprises such as civil engineering projects or assembly-line manufacturing. The resource management type of project team is oriented towards projects fortunate enough to have well defined and tangible goals which are resource limited rather than intellect limited.

Neither the scientist-intensive system nor the resource management system employ a collective, multidisciplinary knowledge to establish an optimal research mentality. Both systems try to make the new drug application a tangible and well-defined goal from the outset. Unfortunately, the goals of a research-oriented industry are not generally as tangible or definable as goals in non-research environments. Rather, the goals tend to be conceptual and are often phrased as hypotheses.

The solution to this conflict may be to redefine the mission of project teams to predominantly scientific research goals which are, by their nature, hypothesis oriented and intellect limited. The critical-mass based system of clinical drug development incorporates such goals. The *critical mass approach* (Figure 4) performs an interdisciplinary coordination function, as do the scientist-intensive and resource management types of project teams. However, the mechanisms used to coordinate projects are obviously different among these three approaches. Moreover, the critical mass approach creates a continuum in the drug development process by fostering interactions among all of the disciplines participating on the project team. The critical mass research team is charged with the responsibility of developing and sustaining an optimal research mentality. Each of the disciplines represented on the team must nurture the formation of project-associated critical masses within their specific areas of expertise. Thus, continuity of the critical mass research team is not easily perturbed since it promotes a desirable minimal level of redundancy by fostering a collective research mentality. With this redundancy, loss of any team member is not likely to impair the critical mass nature of the project team. Therefore, the project team can progress toward attainment of short-term goals (e.g., NDA) and development of long-term corporate research goals (e.g., research equity).

IV. WHY IS CRITICAL MASS ESSENTIAL?

It is vital to review the essential nature of critical mass. Our fundamental guiding principle throughout this book is that the drug development process functions to determine the benefit/risk profile for an investigational drug. The process of benefit/risk assessment consists of two main components. First, substantial evidence must be accumulated to show that the drug is safe and effective in its intended use, as required by the Federal Food, Drug and Cosmetic Act [7]:

> Sec. 505 [355]. (a) No person shall introduce or deliver for introduction into interstate commerce any new drug, unless an approval of an application filed pursuant to subsection (b) is effective with respect to such drug. (b) Any person may file with the Secretary an application with respect to any drug subject to the provisions of subsection (a). Such persons shall submit to the Secretary as a part of the application (1) full reports of the investigations which have been made to show whether or not such drug is safe for use and whether such drug is effective for use;

Second, the benefits associated with the use of this drug must exceed the risks associated with its administration [8]:

> Concisely compare kind and incidence of beneficial experience with kind and incidence of adverse experience found in clinical studies.

Although the process of benefit/risk assessment seems straightforward, the evolving scientific complexity of new drugs and medical practice, along with the four to ten year time period needed to take a new chemical entity from filing an IND to approval of an NDA, dictates a drug development process that is susceptible to numerous breeches in continuity. Numerous examples of such breaks in continuity have been listed in the previous chapter. Breaks in continuity have varying impact on drug development programs, including disruptions of minor inconvenience, delayed drug development, increased cost of drug development, or rendering a clinical trial program non-supportive with respect to drug approval.

In an effort to delineate approaches toward minimization of such discontinuities, *research mentality* has been described as the intellectual basis for continuity in drug development [9]. Operationally, research mentality with respect to development of specific new chemical entities would be exercised by a multidisciplinary research team comprising a *critical mass*. Critical mass is that property of a research team provided by the presence of several interactive and mutually catalytic scientists who function collectively to produce a dynamic research intellect. The integrity of purpose of the critical mass project team is derived from its mission to construct, sustain, exploit, and increase the research mentality. The importance of critical mass for achievement of intellectual advances in industrial America, as well as in the pharmaceutical industry, has been discussed by Kanter [10] and Bartholini [11]. Clinical drug development via a critical mass research team is capable of attaining the short-term goal of drug approval and facilitating long-term research that is both scientifically progressive and commercially profitable. Thus, implementation of a critical mass-based approach to drug development will facilitate attainment of research mentality, continuity, and research equity.

V. RESEARCH EQUITY

Research equity is defined as the cumulative knowledge possessed by the collective corporate research mentality in a specific area of therapeutic drug research. Research equity is the portion of the corporate research mentality that must be retained to form the foundation for further drug development and innovation, thereby increasing return on the intellectual investment. This equity can be thought of as the value of research mentality over and above its contribution to the specific project for which research was performed. Research equity is typified by preclinical research teams that work cooperatively to exploit a collective knowledge in order to discover and evaluate new chemical entities.

This concept of accumulation of research equity over time is analogous to the concepts involved in the time value of money. Which dollar would you choose: $1 today or $1 that I will give you in ten years? Of course, $1 received in ten years is worth less than $1 today because money has time value. Therefore, you would choose $1 today. Hence, a person will only defer current consumption if his invested money grows in value. Money invested at *simple* interest only earns interest on the invested principal. For example, $1000 deposited in a savings account with 8% annual simple interest will grow by $80 per year, i.e., the account value will be $1080 after one year, $1160 after two years, $1240 after three years, and $3400 after 30 years. Contrast this simple interest situation with money invested at *compound* interest. With compounding, interest is added to the account at the end of the year, then the combined principal plus interest becomes the beginning balance that earns interest for the next year. For example, $1000 deposited in the savings account with 8% annual compound interest will grow to $1080 in one year, $1166.40 after two years, $1259.71 after three years, and $10,062.66 after 30 years! With compounding, the long-term value after 30 years in this example is almost triple the value with simple interest. In research, the accumulation of knowledge as research equity is analogous to growth of knowledge with compound interest, not simple interest, because the interest over time is growing based on both the original knowledge (the principal) plus the new knowledge acquired in past years (the interest). This compounding of interest leads to the ever-increasing size of our knowledge base over time; this growing knowledge base is our equity in the research process. Similar to other financial strategies, research equity can be left in a given project to continue to grow or transferred as an investment in other projects. The notion of transferable research equity is discussed later in this chapter.

Progressing a drug from the chemist's bench to the marketplace does not in itself assure a corporation of increased research equity. A group of scientists performing their individual tasks sequentially will not form the dynamic, intellect-expanding critical mass which is the basis of research equity. Research equity accrues to the corporation when critical mass project teams develop a *sustained* intellect and research mentality.

In contrast with preclinical research, the clinical drug development program generally does not foster formation of research equity. Clinical development of a new compound may be executed by two or three independent groups of clinical scientists: the clinical pharmacology group, a Phase II/III clinical trials group, and a post-marketing research group. Depending upon the organizational structure of the company, it is typical that no clinical scientist will be involved in all three of these segments of clinical drug development. Consequently, changes are needed in such conventional clinical drug development methods in order to build contributions by clinical research personnel to corporate research equity.

VI. ADAPTATIONS IN PROJECT MANAGEMENT TO INCORPORATE CRITICAL MASS

Two major philosophical adaptations must be made in conventional project management systems to render them a source of accruing research equity. First, and probably most important, the project team must be given the responsibility for accomplishing a research-oriented conceptual goal, namely, development of the optimal research mentality concerning a given drug development project. Such conceptual goals are much more rational for activities that are intellect limited rather than resource limited.

Second, the project team must be comprised of a critical mass rather than a resource management structure alone. Moreover, the project team must foster the formation of smaller critical masses within each of the areas of expertise represented on the team. These critical masses across all project teams in the company must form a collective intellectual and experiential resource which is dynamic and self-sustaining. A properly constituted critical mass will assure establishment of a certain minimal redundancy such that several scientists included in the critical mass understand any given aspect of the research mentality housed by that team. Thus, a critical mass has minimal sensitivity to alterations in its composition so long as those compositional alterations do not reduce the research mass below a critical level.

This type of project management would promote achievement of a drug development continuum involving project team members from the time of drug discovery until optimal knowledge of the compound has been achieved. Thus, a collective mentality would be available for all aspects of the drug development process. While the specific expertise of project team members dictates that each would be primarily responsible for various practical tasks, the team as a whole would be responsible for producing viable products and, consequently, must be oriented toward collecting any available information that might facilitate development or discovery of new chemical entities in that therapeutic area.

We have emphasized that each of the contributory disciplines that participate in the project team must assemble separate critical masses. By nurturing and including a series of expertise-specific critical masses within the project team, the research team is assured of comprising a multidisciplinary critical mass. In addition, changes within any given segment of research are unlikely to perturb the overall critical mass of the project team. Thus, preservation and evolution of the research mentality is facilitated, as is growth of research equity. Without formation of a critical mass, the creativity encompassed in a given research project will be limited in part by the creativity of the least creative scientist working independently on the new compound.

VII. OBSTACLES TO FORMATION OF CRITICAL MASS PROJECT TEAMS

Avots [12] compiled an important publication on the main reasons project management fails. These observations were made across a variety of industries, including the pharmaceutical industry. Although it was published over 20 years ago, the principles are still clearly applicable today. Project management fails because the basis for the project is not sound, the wrong person was appointed project manager, corporate management is not supportive, project parameters are inadequately defined, management techniques are misused, and termination of the project is not planned (Table 2). Based on these observations, Avots [12] offered ten lessons for success in utilizing project management (Table 3). This work on general causes of failure and resulting lessons is applicable to the pharmaceutical industry. However, in addition to these general concepts, there are other factors specific to the pharmaceutical industry that must be considered.

Table 2. Listing of the most common reasons for failure of project management.

1. basis for the project is not sound
2. wrong person appointed project manager
   - project manager must be an organizer and leader
   - project manager must recognize the continuous trade-off conflict between costs, schedules, and technical performance
   - project manager must be capable of effective arbitration
   - project manager must not become preoccupied with any single aspect of the project
3. lack of strong support from company management
4. inadequate definitions of project objectives, work content, cost, schedule, and technical requirements
   - formalized task statements must exist to specify the role of each contributor
   - develop contingency plans to enable rapid response to problems that can be anticipated
5. misuse of management techniques
   - over-reliance on excessively sophisticated computerized management tools (e.g., PERT or Gantt charts)
   - greatest need is for easily comprehensible manual planning techniques and simple user-oriented reports
6. lack of planning of project termination
   - project team members often see the completion of the project as a threat due to uncertainty of future assignments

Source: Ref. 12

Three major inter-related obstacles arise in the pharmaceutical industry to obstruct formation of critical mass project teams. First, scientists with different expertise must be encouraged to interact and learn to communicate in order to form critical masses. Second, personnel with expertise in drug development must be combined with personnel having expertise in a pharmacotherapeutic specialty, pharmaceutical sciences, or management. Third, and in some respects the thorniest issue, a system of rewards for team members must be developed to promote and recognize the contributions of individuals to the team product, without promoting isolated individual effort. Clearly, the means to overcome these three obstacles must be corporation specific. However, a few general comments may be useful.

The multidisciplinary nature of the drug development process can be a barrier to effective communication due to discipline-specific terminology. In addition, effective communication may be impeded by scientists who are specialized to the exclusion of general knowledge or interest in other

Table 3. Major lessons for success in project management.

1. When starting project management, plan to go all the way. It is best to initiate with full project managers and not settle for less authority with project coordinators.
2. Do not skimp on the project manager's qualifications.
3. Do not spare time and effort in laying out the project groundwork and defining work.
4. Insure that work packages in the project are of the proper size.
5. Establish and use network planning techniques, having the network as the focal point of project implementation.
6. Be sure the information flow related to the project management system is realistic.
7. Be prepared to continually replan jobs to accommodate frequent changes on dynamic projects.
8. Whenever possible, tie together responsibility, performance, and rewards. Identify the channels for resolving conflicts.
9. Long before a project ends, provide some means for accommodating the employees' personal goals.
10. If mistakes in project implementation have been made, make a fresh try.

Source: Ref. 12.

areas. Achievement of effective and efficient communication is a major challenging prerequisite to formation and success of a critical mass project team in complex organizations [13]. The need for effective, efficient communication and management at the boundaries among the project team and other parties in the organization have been stressed as essential precursors of successful team performance in the pharmaceutical industry and other R&D enterprises [14-16]. Promoting discussion of project-related scientific information may be one means of overcoming the communication problem since that information should be a common interest of all project team members.

Unfortunately, fostering generalized interest among expertise-specific groups is not accomplished simply by including personnel with some interdisciplinary interests on the team. The combination of personnel who form a team must include personnel with expertise in drug development and personnel with expertise in the specific pharmacotherapeutic area of research. The balance of these two principal types of personnel for any specific project will be determined by the unique characteristics of that project. Few generalizations can be made as to the personnel needs of different drug development projects; however, it is unreasonable to expect a single scientist to possess knowledge of the drug development process, expertise in the pharmacotherapeutic specialty, sufficient knowledge of the other contributory disciplines, and the managerial prowess required for the project team. Cost-effective and expeditious clinical drug development requires a project team with input from multiple individuals in order to establish a dynamic, catalytic combination of pharmacotherapeutic expertise, drug development knowledge, and interdisciplinary understanding.

Rewards for contributions to a project team must include monetary compensation, as well as opportunities to further develop research interests. While financial rewards are desirable, many scientists value personal opportunities as highly desirable and include this opportunity factor as a consideration in long-term career plans [12,17]. Assignments to desirable projects and receipt of financial rewards must be delivered in a way that encourages continued team participation and team productivity, rather than encouraging isolated individual effort.

VIII. SUMMARY

The need for coordination in pharmaceutical corporations is obvious. The pharmaceutical industry, at least on the non-generic side, is research intensive. Indeed, successful invention sustains the innovative pharmaceutical industry. Research and development activities consume a disproportionately large portion of corporate resources due in part to the diversity of opportunity for product development and the multidisciplinary nature of drug development. A pharmaceutical corporation must simultaneously finance multiple research activities in diverse areas such as cardiovascular products, infectious disease, and psychopharmacology. Since research activity in and of itself can not produce a profit, the manufacturing and sales segments of the industry must be coordinated with other diversified activities in order for a company to be profitable. As discussed, manufacturing and sales' activities are amenable to the tangible goal orientation of conventional project management to optimize cost-effectiveness and productivity. If for no other reason than simplicity, it is appealing to corporate management to apply these same project management tools to research and development activities. While a project management system can be established for research and development, its focus and operation must be different from that used in manufacturing and sales in order to recognize that research and development goals are hypothesis oriented and intellect limited, rather than goal oriented and resource limited. Research and development project teams must be constructed as a multidisciplinary critical mass in order to minimize vulnerability to breaks in continuity and inadequate research mentality, as well as to optimize development of research equity.

Research equity has two notable features that sustain and grow the experience base and intellectual mass of the corporation. First, a portion of research equity can be recycled into other research projects within the same therapeutic area. That is, the project team can re-utilize their expertise in development of other drugs. It must be cautioned, however, that this recycled research equity is only available as long as a critical mass is sustained within a given area of therapeutic drug research.

The second notable feature of research equity is that a portion of research equity is transferable to research projects that are not obviously related to the original source of research equity. This transferable equity concerns knowledge of the drug development process, rather than knowledge unique to a specific pharmacotherapeutic area. For example, a person who successfully participated in clinical development of an antidepressant drug should have learned general concepts of drug development that would be valuable to a new project on an anti-inflammatory agent. Such transferable equity further increases opportunity for return on intellectual investment. The transferable portion of research equity and the personnel who will carry that research equity in the transfer can be utilized to spawn new critical masses in new areas of research. Thus, the acquisition and judicious allocation of research equity can have far reaching impact on the long-term productivity and profitability of a corporation. Failure to acquire research equity or failure to appreciate its importance will favor adoption of a short-term mentality resulting in frequent breaks in continuity and suboptimal product development. Consequently, even very good compounds will fail to achieve their optimal success in the marketplace and corporations investing large sums of money in research will have limited opportunities for return on investment.

On a practical note, one must realize the tremendous challenge of assembling and managing a research organization comprised of critical mass project teams. Such an organization is highly dependent upon its ability to hire and retain quality personnel, as well as the corporation's ability to invest some resources solely for the long term. In general, progress by a critical mass research team will be determined by the most creative intellects on the team. Some combination of compensation and professional opportunities must be used to attract creative and productive scientists. Other authors have written extensively on the managerial environment essential to discovery and new product development [17-21]. Selected comments from Deming are provided in Table 4. Creative scientists will be attracted to an opportunity to build research equity. The transferable nature of research equity offers research administration a device to help project teams that are not optimally productive. In addition, the critical mass project team structure will accommodate reassignment of personnel and research equity to other related and unrelated areas of drug development without ravaging the source projects.

Table 4. Selected comments from W. Edwards Deming on management.

1. Individualistic competition undermines the intrinsic motivation and teamwork essential for success.
2. Motivation and leadership must be aligned with money, machines, and techniques.
3. Design and build fireproof systems rather than spend time fighting fires.
4. People must be encouraged to excel and to continue to learn.
5. People are entitled to have fun, to have joy in learning and work.

Source: Ref. 21

The administrative team which oversees the critical mass project system must itself be a critical mass comprised of senior research executives. This research management critical mass can then allocate resources and transferable research equity to address the research priorities of the corporation needed to foster optimal research mentality and productivity.

Of course, observers will insist on some measure of the success or failure of such an approach to clinical drug development. At present, it is difficult to identify a standard by which pharmaceutical research productivity can be measured or judged as optimal. Teitelman and Baldo [22] devised a composite index based on total R&D expenditure versus total new product sales over the 1980s decade. While this index does provide one way to compare companies, only their own survey used the index to date. For want of a better yardstick, one might use the historical success rate of approximately 1 in 10,000 new chemical entities making it to market [23]. It is tempting to believe that a careful, thoughtful, interactive drug discovery and development continuum with research equity can produce a higher success rate because it will exploit a greater research mentality than is the current predominant practice. In a profit-motivated industry, a higher success rate is desirable. However, the commitment to the acquisition and management of research equity requires a long-term approach to research and development and to personnel within the research organization.

REFERENCES

1. Obligations of sponsors and monitors of clinical investigations. *Federal Register* Volume 42 (Number 187): 49612–49630 (September 27, 1977).
2. Obligations of clinical investigators of regulated articles. *Federal Register* Volume 43 (Number 153): 35210–35236 (August 8, 1978).
3. Protection of human subjects; informed consent. *Federal Register* Volume 46 (Number 17): 8942–8980 (January 27, 1981).

4. New drug and antibiotic regulations. *Federal Register* Volume 50 (Number 36): 7452–7519 (February 22, 1985).

5. New drug, antibiotic, and biologic drug product regulations; final rule. *Federal Register* Volume 52 (number 53): 8798–8847 (1987).

6. Cocchetto DM, Nardi RV. Benefit-risk assessment of investigational drugs: current methodology, limitations, and alternative approaches. *Pharmacotherapy* 6: 286–303 (1986).

7. *Federal Food, Drug and Cosmetic Act*. Washington, D.C.: U.S. Government Printing Office, 1979.

8. Title 21, *Code of Federal Regulations*, article 314.1. Washington, D.C.: U.S. Government Printing Office, 1980, page 94.

9. Cocchetto DM, Nardi RV. Challenges to maintaining continuity through expanded clinical trials and the approval period. In: *Clinical Trials and Tribulations* (Cato AE, editor). New York: Marcel Dekker, Inc., 1988, pp. 253–274.

10. Kanter RM. *The Change Masters*. New York: Simon & Schuster, 1983.

11. Bartholini G. Organization of industrial drug research. In: *Decision Making in Drug Research* (Gross F, ed.). New York: Raven Press, pp. 123–146, 1983.

12. Avots I. Why does project management fail? *California Management Review* 12 (Number 1): 77–82 (1969).

13. Conrad C. *Strategic Organizational Communication*. New York: Holt, Rinehart and Winston, 1985.

14. Conrad C. Barriers to communication in complex pharmaceutical organizations. *Clin. Res. Practices and Drug Reg. Affairs* 4: 485–509 (1986).

15. Heininger SA. R&D and competitiveness—what leaders must do. *Research Technology Management*, pp. 6–7, November–December 1988.

16. Ancona DG, Caldwell D. Improving the performance of new product teams. *Research Technology Management*, pp. 25–29, March–April 1990.

17. Root-Bernstein RS. Who discovers and invents. *Research Technology Management*, pp.43–50, January–February 1989.

18. Root-Bernstein RS. Strategies of research. *Research Technology Management*, pp. 36–41, May–June 1989.

19. Root-Bernstein RS. *Discovering*. Cambridge, MA: Harvard University Press, 1989.

20. Deming WE. *Out of the Crisis*. Cambridge, MA: MIT Center for Advanced Engineering Study, 1986.

21. Macoby M. Deming critiques american management. *Research Technology Management*, pp. 43–44, May–June 1990.

22. Teitelman R, Baldo A. Which companies in the drug business get their money's worth out of research spending? Grading R&D. *Financial World*, pp. 22–24 (January 24, 1989).

23. Reuben BG, Wittcoff HA. *Pharmaceutical Chemicals in Perspective*. New York: John Wiley & Sons, 1989, page 33.

9

Resource-Limited Versus Intellect-Limited Projects

Research is not a
timeclock-monkey-wrench job.

Martin H. Fischer

I. INTRODUCTION

Many companies in the pharmaceutical industry, as well as other industries, began to use various project management systems in the 1970s and 1980s. The pharmaceutical industry began to explore these systems in an effort to achieve greater coordination among activities of the multidisciplinary departments contributing to the drug development process. Unfortunately, some managers overlooked the fact that some project management systems were developed in the construction, engineering, and aerospace industries as a means to facilitate completion of projects that were rate limited by availability of resources in a certain timed sequence. For construction, consider the simple example that architectural work must be completed before the superstructure is erected and the superstructure must precede electrical contracting. This type of project is known as a resource-limited project. Increased resources, e.g., more manpower or equipment, would hasten completion of the project.

The second type of project is an intellect-limited project. In these projects, completion of the project is rate limited by availability of knowledge. For example, current developments of biotechnology products (e.g., human insulin, tissue plasminogen activator) depended on intellectual breakthroughs in understanding the fundamental structure and function of nucleic acids, as well as the biochemistry of proteins. Such projects will be facilitated by an intellectual advance, but not necessarily by supplemental resources.

This chapter explores the differences between resource-limited projects and intellect-limited projects. These differences are considered in some detail because project managers must be able to characterize their projects as either resource- or intellect-limited. Further, some project management systems are useful management tools only for resource-limited projects. Finally, the more business-driven side of most pharmaceutical companies (i.e., manufacturing, marketing, and sales divisions) typically functions as resource-limited operations, while the R&D side of most pharmaceutical companies typically functions as intellect-limited operations. Some understanding of these different rate-limiting factors in different parts of the company is an essential precursor to considering the research-marketing interface, i.e., the topic of the next chapter.

II. CHARACTERISTICS OF RESOURCE-LIMITED VERSUS INTELLECT-LIMITED PROJECTS

The pharmaceutical industry, particularly research-driven innovator companies, faces a major challenge to coordinate their income generation (from the efforts of manufacturing, marketing, and sales) with use of part of this income to generate new products from their research and development efforts. Income results directly from manufacturing, marketing, and sales. These income-generating activities can be summarized as a catalytic process of combining capital, manpower, a product knowledge base, and a plan in order to achieve a saleable product. In general, the knowledge base on the product remains relatively constant in the short term. Hence, the plan to utilize that information remains fairly constant since the creativity of the plan is limited by the realities of the knowledge base on the drug. Modifications of the plan usually represent changes that do not increase the total content of the plan. That is, some part of the old plan is replaced by a newer, more efficient information-utilizing component. Output from resource-limited projects is not dramatically affected by changes in the knowledge base or plan that do not involve substantial growth in total information content. The resource-limited nature of some sales activity is indicated by the fact that sales for many drugs increase with increases in capital expenditure and manpower (e.g., sales personnel). For example, the concordance between sales and "detail calls" for certain antibiotics is evidence of a classic resource-limited situation. Examples of resource-limited projects come from the construction industry and military rapid-deployment operations. One implication for resource-limited projects is that output can be maintained during periods of personnel deficits via addition of capital resources to the project. The basic characteristics of resource-limited projects are summarized in Table 1.

The resource-limited situation is in sharp contrast to the activities and processes that are necessary to produce and sustain viable research and development. R&D activities can be summarized as a catalytic process of combining capital, manpower, and a plan in order to produce a knowledge base (i.e., research equity). This statement emphasizes that the product of research is the knowledge base on the product or, as we have previously defined, research equity. This case is an intellect-limited situation and the intellect resides within the personnel who are participating in the project (Table 1). In this case, the plan is constantly changing due to feedback modification from the growing knowledge base, which resides within the personnel participating in the project. Similarly, the personnel are also

Table 1. Comparison of the major characteristics of resource-limited and intellect-limited projects.

	Resource-Limited Projects	Intellect-Limited Projects
Output	dollars or product	information
Use of capital	quantity of output is directly proportional to capital	quality (not quantity) of output may be increased via capital investment
Information	an essential input to the project; total information content of project team is relatively constant	information is the output
Plan	plan may become more efficient; plan is often static; scope of the plan may change, but rarely expands	plan is dynamic; scope can expand or contract as needed
Personnel	output is directly proportional to quantity of personnel (man-days)	output is directly proportional to the intellectual pace (research mentality) of personnel
Timeframe	highly predictable; well suited to PERT charts and Gantt methods	uncertain; poorly suited to PERT or Gantt methods
Inputs	capital, personnel, plan, information	capital, plan, personnel

altered as a result of the impact of new information on their collective research mentality. In contrast with resource-limited projects, personnel deficits on an intellect-limited project can not be compensated by addition of capital resources to the project. Manipulating capital resources generally will have little, if any, positive impact on the production of information, at least in the short term. Capital investment generally improves efficiency, but will not have a multiplicative effect on yield of new knowledge. In fact, capital investment is more necessary to retain state of the art capabilities and, thereby, the quality of information, rather than quantitatively improving output of information.

Consider the effects of adding new personnel to an intellect-limited project. Addition of new personnel who are unfamiliar with the R&D project may actually impair the yield of knowledge, at least until these new personnel become integrated into the critical mass project team. Interestingly, new project personnel may actually add new ideas and spawn new projects, at least initially, rather than improve the speed with which an existing project and existing ideas are progressed. Consequently, the R&D manager of intellect-limited projects must spend considerable time evaluating the intellectual pace of his personnel by evaluating their research plans. This managerial focus contrasts sharply with a manager of resource-limited activities, who can focus the evaluation on capital investment and personnel (i.e., man-days) based on production of either a product or dollars.

An important and subtle concept is that the R&D manager must be able to evaluate the quality of *negative* information (e.g., a study failing to show any differences between drug and placebo), as well as positive information, obtained in any research effort. This negative information is vital to justifiable decisions to terminate projects that are highly unlikely to be successful or in directing efforts in a given multifaceted project towards a particular achievable goal on the road to overall project success. Since each successful drug development project is accompanied by many unsuccessful projects, R&D managers must be adept at making proper and rapid decisions based on both positive and negative studies.

III. CONSIDERATIONS FOR MANAGING INTELLECT-LIMITED PROJECTS

The pharmaceutical industry is highly dependent on productive research for innovation and new products. However, the immediate consequence of research is expenses. Research contributes to current income only indirectly through such factors as enhancing the company's scientific reputation and credibility. Research must always be viewed as a long-term investment; therein lies the challenge. Since income from new products is required to sustain the vitality of any company, research projects that appear to have promise must be coordinated with activities related to the ultimate ability of this project to generate direct income. This coordination is essential in light of the long period of time required to move a new product through the research, development, and regulatory processes to the marketplace.

Unfortunately, the drug development process has become a victim of the vocabulary used to describe it. Commonly, research divisions in the pharmaceutical industry are labeled "Research and Development." For reasons that only history can probably clarify, products that have entered clinical trials in humans are considered "in development" and everything else is considered "in research." Actually, the entire drug development process is a research activity, with the major emphasis being placed on an information-gathering, knowledge-expanding effort. In fact, drug development is more rationally divided into discovery research and development research. Discovery research efforts concentrate on identifying disease processes susceptible to pharmacological intervention, identifying moieties capable of altering physiologic activities, and generating new chemical entities with pharmacologic activity. Structure-activity evaluations are vital to the characterization of new chemical entities. Such evaluations are actually a developmental exercise in the sense that a novel activity has already been discovered and, even if it could be improved, it would still have known pharmacologic activity.

Structure-activity characterizations cannot be factored into schedules that avoid impacting the resource-limited side of the company, namely, manufacturing, marketing, and sales. It is similarly short sighted to fix the clinical research program and rigidly schedule the time course of clinical research in the absence of a clear understanding of the pharmacologic and toxicologic profile of a new chemical entity in humans. Such short-sighted approaches trivialize the clinical drug development process into a regulatory hurdle-jumping exercise. For an aggressive and intellectually viable drug development program, the focus must remain on developing optimal knowledge about the compound that has been selected to become the company's new product. This is not to say that the clinical drug development process or the whole development process, for that matter, should be an unfocused research exercise. Rather, R&D should be directed towards optimizing the knowledge base that resides within the critical mass research team. Efforts in this direction are generally not resource-limited. As discussed previously, generation of an optimal research mentality by a critical mass research team generates research equity for the project team and the corporation.

The effort to accrue research equity can be affected by resources allocated to the project. However, this is not simply a "more is better" situation. As we have discussed, merely increasing personnel and expenditures for intellect-limited projects is not a mechanism to guarantee increased production of knowledge that will advance the project. Careful, almost experimental, additions of resources to an intellect-limited project is the preferred approach by R&D management. Of course, wholesale disruption of a critical mass research team has consequences. A productive team could be destroyed without any guarantee that a new productive critical mass would be re-established after re-allocation of personnel. In fact, it is probably almost impossible to achieve short-term increases in research productivity without sacrificing longer-term productivity of some aspects of the research organization. Dynamic resource allocation from a small, select group of flexible reserves to a project, rather than permanent commitments of more manpower to empire-building projects, is a means to provide adequate manpower without disrupting the long-term maintenance of critical mass. Thus, the leadership of research organizations must be able to (1) assess whether research plans will produce the desired scientific information, (2) foster establishment of critical mass research teams, and (3) be sensitive to the retention of critical mass research activities as personnel changes are made.

10

Interactions Between Clinical Research and Marketing Groups

Every one lives by selling something.

Robert Louis Stevenson

I. INTRODUCTION

Previous chapters have focused principally on project-oriented issues that must be considered by management to optimize the knowledge gained in clinical research. We have described the challenges involved in organizing a project and assembling critical mass research teams. We have argued that research teams function as the corporation's means to generate both project-specific knowledge and project non-specific research equity for the corporation.

We have also addressed the challenges that research management must meet in an attempt to optimize research productivity. Clear and important distinctions were made between intellect-limited and resource-limited projects. The critical differences between intellect-limited projects (typically conducted in preclinical research and clinical research) and resource-limited projects (generally associated with the income-producing segments of the pharmaceutical industry, i.e., production and sales) must be factored into senior management's decision-making process. We will now turn our attention to the primary challenge for research management, namely, integration of the overall research program with the income-producing efforts of the company. This is one of the major challenges for any corporation with activity in both research and marketing.

II. MARKET-PUSH VERSUS RESEARCH-PULL AS THE BASIS OF INNOVATION

It has become quite fashionable over the last few years to characterize a successful business as market driven. Peters and Waterman [1] popularized the notion of market-driven, customer-conscious companies. This notion has been embraced by some pharmaceutical company executives [2]. In fact, some research organizations have boasted of their efforts to engage in market-driven basic research. We will argue in this chapter that market-driven research yields only "me too" products (i.e., patented generic drugs), rather than innovative therapeutic advances. This concept of bounded yield of market-driven research is the genesis of the argument that the discovery of important research questions and the potential for developing clinically important new therapies arise from information gained in the research community long before the marketplace notices the importance of the area of research. We presented information in Chapter 1 to show that significant therapeutic advances are the result of new understanding about a disease or the approach to treating it.

The limitations of market-driven research can be seen easier after introducing terminology. We distinguish between "market push" and "research pull" as sources of innovation. Figure 1 illustrates the anchoring of marketing-based approaches in historical information, thereby necessitating that marketing push from the past toward the future with limited vision of future technologies. The limitations of market-based information in predicting compounds of importance in the future were cited by Reidenberg [3]. In contrast, the research-pull approach is anchored in development of new future technologies which comprise the vision toward which the present is pulled. Innovative developments from research-pull approaches have as part of their character some decidedly non-linear intellectual accomplishments.

The limitations of market-push research may be best illustrated by a common approach used to identify research projects with perceived high market value. A pharmaceutical company's market research department would assemble a set of questionnaires designed to solicit information about unmet needs or opportunities that exist either across the whole medical

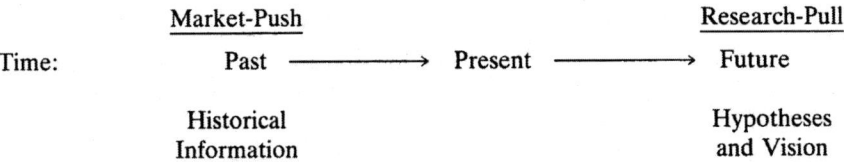

Figure 1. Market-push vs. research-pull as sources of innovation.

profession or in a selected sub-specialty. These questionnaires would be administered, probably in a focus group format, to a group of physicians who would respond based on their professional experience and knowledge. Analysis of their responses is purported to show "market identified unmet needs." In such settings, physicians identify (1) the shortcomings of existing therapies and (2) inadequately treated subsets of patients. Market research equates these two types of physician-identified deficiencies in current practice to "unmet needs." For example, physicians may report that the frequency of sexual dysfunction with several marketed antihypertensive agents is an important shortcoming of those drugs. Subsequently, market research would infer that a desirable property of a new antihypertensive drug is the absence of sexual dysfunction. As another example, physicians may report that a large group of depressed patients are not treated adequately with currently marketed antidepressants. Therefore, market research would infer that development of new antidepressants is a fruitful general disease target. Findings of the first type may lead to new products with modified properties, but not properties dramatically different from current therapies. Findings of the second type are based on information that has long been known in the research community. Consequently, the opportunities identified by the market place are actually opportunities that have been known for an extended period of time in the research community.

A given physician's perception of the importance of a disease will depend on the size of the patient population, as well as published reports on medical and pharmacologic research for the disease. A few examples will illustrate this point. Reports of dementia date back to antiquity, as do reports of tumors, ulcers, obstructive airways disease, and a host of other diseases that have become the focus of much research in this century. On an individual disease basis, the impact of dementia has not changed dramatically over the last 30 years. However, the perception of its importance has changed. Several factors have combined to heighten our perception that development of treatments for this condition warrants investment of significant energy and resources. First, we are witnessing the "graying" of the western world following the baby boom generation. Second, research on Alzheimer's disease, which was originally described for the case of a 51-year-old demented woman in 1907 by Alois Alzheimer [4,5], has provided insight into some of the mechanisms that may be associated with pathological manifestations of brain dysfunction and atrophy, common manifestations of the aging process. Similarly, work on other neurodegenerative diseases has not ruled out the hypothesis that senility and Alzheimer's disease may be the result of premature aging of the brain and, therefore, may not actually represent pathologies that are treatable. Over the last several decades, basic research on the anatomy and physiology of neurodegenerative diseases is responsible for our perception that these diseases present an immeasurable opportunity for drug development. We do not mean to imply that scientists understand enough to enable highly focused drug development that will surely be successful in treating this disease. However, researchers in this area and those with an active interest in drug development do not need a market research survey to identify this target as an important drug development target. Dementia was identified as a research-pull target long ago.

Consequently, if a corporation has developed their research division appropriately, an insightful analysis of unmet needs could be conducted in 30–40 minute interviews with one-half dozen of the researchers within the company and through similar interviews with a few medical research physicians. In fact, a relatively simple literature survey is likely to identify areas of opportunity just as effectively as a "market needs" analysis conducted by a conventional market research group.

An even more dangerous aspect of "needs analysis" is that these analyses may be used to set the corporation's research priorities [3]. We must live with the reality that the marketing analyses will only provide information in response to the specific questions asked and only where a historical database exists. This may or may not provide an adequate perspective on the potential to develop a new drug in a given therapeutic area. Similarly, this may or may not provide an adequate perspective on the financial rewards of a successful drug development effort in a given therapeutic area. Recent history is strewn with illusions of market financial projections that ultimately bore little relationship to the realities of marketed drugs. Cimetidine was initially thought to be a competitor for antacids. When Sir James Black was working to identify a selective histamine antagonist, Smith Kline & French (SKF) was wrestling with whether or not this endeavor had a sufficient market potential to make its investment worthwhile. Had SKF appreciated that H-2-antagonists would represent a $2+ billion annual U.S. market some 15 years after the introduction of cimetidine, any discussion about terminating this research endeavor would have been unlikely. It is noteworthy that occurrences throughout the 1970s and 1980s at SKF demonstrated clearly the 8–10 year time lag for observing the consequences of strategic research decisions [6]. Interestingly, the antacid market continues to be quite unperturbed by the availability of several H-2-antagonists. Similarly, the OTC antihistamine/decongestant market continues to grow despite availability in the last few years of prescription nonsedating antihistamines.

Minoxidil provides another example of poor research prioritization made in part on the basis of conventional marketing information. Projections of a large market potential for minoxidil for treatment of male pattern baldness drove The Upjohn Company and investors to invest heavily in development of this compound. Unfortunately, the high expectations have not been met. These are only two of the many examples that could be cited. Clearly, conventional market research has the potential to dramatically underestimate market potential (e.g., cimetidine) and dramatically overestimate market potential (e.g., minoxidil).

This discussion is not meant to imply that market research is a worthless endeavor, nor is it our contention that marketing should not attempt to evaluate the market potential of research compounds. Market research can facilitate identification of opportunities for line extension products or me-too compounds. However, market research has limited value in the decision-making process of directing the corporate research program. Rather, the corporate research program should be directed in full view of the talents, background, and experience of the members of the research team. These individuals have the ability both to identify unmet medical needs and know the therapeutic targets which their capabilities can best address. The combination of these two items provides the foundation for innovative clinical drug development.

III. INTERACTION BETWEEN RESEARCH AND MARKETING

We argued in a previous chapter that excessive marketing control can perturb development of research mentality within any given project. The preceding section of this chapter argues that market-push decisions can perturb the development of research equity within a project and, even more importantly, impair the ability of the research operation to develop new therapeutic advances. It seems paradoxical to suggest that market-push research can reduce the return on investment in R&D, but that can be the case. This paradox has fueled conflict between R&D and marketing personnel in many companies. It is important to examine this conflict.

R&D and marketing personnel must communicate effectively. The competitive environment of rapid changes in the marketplace and the high cost of product development make effective communication essential. The conflict often begins when R&D managers look to marketing to prepare plans to launch new products, while many marketing personnel want R&D to invent new products with certain desirable characteristics. The resistance of R&D managers to marketing information has been systematically studied. Gupta and Wilemon [7] surveyed 80 R&D managers across a variety of technology-intensive companies regarding their use of marketing information. Seventy-five percent of R&D managers perceived the biggest problem as a lack of understanding on the part of marketing managers of product design trade-offs. In addition, 66% of R&D managers thought that marketing reports contained too many unsupported generalizations. Perhaps most interestingly, 50% of R&D managers said marketing information reflected a limited understanding of customer needs! This last finding is indicative of the conflict between what we call the research-pull perspective versus a marketing-push perspective.

Concern about marketing-based perturbations in R&D was reflected in the R&D managers thoughts that marketing managers believe in forcing their views on R&D and marketing managers do not understand the process of new product development. In this study, R&D managers were specifically asked why they resist using marketing information. The portion of R&D managers citing the top three reasons for not using marketing information was as follows: incomplete information from marketing (72%), inaccurate information (49%), and marketing's lack of technical competence (35%). These reasons are similar to those cited in earlier work by Deshpande and Zaltman [8].

These supporting observations from studies of a variety of technology-based companies argue that a competitive advantage will belong to the company that can improve mutual understanding and cooperative product development across R&D and marketing personnel. The first and most important aspect of improved understanding is to end the traditional power struggle. It is neither necessary nor desirable that Marketing dominate R&D or that R&D dominate Marketing. In fact, the Marketing and R&D divisions should be independent. In today's pharmaceutical industry, it is miopic to function with the belief that the Marketing group must sell the new chemical entities coming from the R&D group or that R&D should focus their discovery and development efforts according to Marketing's wish list. Each group has more than one avenue to generate profits and knowledge for the corporation. Marketing can introduce new products acquired by licensure efforts. R&D can progress in research by collaborative efforts with specialized research partners. A restrictive viewpoint will create destructive competition and fear of risk; unwillingness to take risk is the door to mediocrity in a research-dependent setting.

The Marketing and R&D groups must learn to collaborate. Each group has expertise that the other needs. As in all collaborations, there will be some times when the groups agree and other times when they disagree. It is not necessary and probably not even possible for the collaboration to include all areas of mutual interest. Those areas in which collaboration seems possible should become the foundation on which to improve communication. The R&D group needs to take the lead in fostering these collaborations because R&D is fundamentally collective and collaborative in nature. To foster collaboration, the R&D group must make itself the source of technical information to the Marketing group. Seizing this initiative is a real opportunity for R&D. This does not mean that R&D should provide volumes of technical reports and hope that someone in Marketing will discern the salient facts. Under such circumstances, Marketing will hire an outside scientific consultant to interpret events with his own unique viewpoint. When Marketing's scientific consultant has an opinion that conflicts with views in R&D, battlelines are drawn and collaboration yields to confrontation. The data become incidental to the argument and any hope for better mutual understanding is ended. Scientists know that such controversies usually arise when two groups attempt to interpret different and incomplete sets of data. Therefore, such situations must be avoided in the interest of building collaboration.

Collaboration and communication can arise from focusing attention on the data. Such a focus can facilitate collaboration because the data are the common item of interest to all parties. The Marketing group must use the data to increase sales of the product, while the R&D personnel are data generators.

Successful collaborations will grow based on mutual respect and an effort to develop a collective and shared information set. Marketing must accept the R&D group as their primary technical consultant and the R&D group must provide that service to the satisfaction of Marketing. Consultants from outside the project team, whether they are within or outside the corporation, must be used to assure that the gaps in technical understanding and research/marketing communications are identified and addressed. Controversies should be settled in light of all available and necessary data, not by opinion or arbitrary decision making. Once the scientific facts are established, Marketing can use the information. Preclinical and clinical scientists interacting with Marketing must be careful to distinquish between data and interpretation in order to minimize confusion in the interaction of R&D and Marketing.

IV. SCOPE OF DISCOVERY RESEARCH: BROAD OR FOCUSED?

A fundamental reality of drug development research is that it will not, by definition, be uniformly successful. In fact, it will more frequently fail than succeed! It is very risky to assume that starting a drug development program with a particular target in mind will ultimately result in the introduction of a drug for that disease. In fact, even "me too" drug development projects do not have a guarantee of success in light of the necessity to find both a safe and effective compound. Moreover, commercial success of the "me too" compound will require at least a minimal scientific or marketing advantage relative to the competition.

Consider the implications of uncertain success for managing a clinical drug development operation. For example, assume that a company's goal is to complete one approvable registration program for a new chemical entity every year. This is indeed an ambitious undertaking. If only 15–25% of all new chemical entities entering clinical evaluation ultimately yield a complete, approvable registration package, 4 to 6 preclinical projects per year must progress to initiation of clinical drug development. If we then back up into the preclinical drug discovery and preclinical development arena, one needs 30 to 100 active preclinical projects to sustain initiation of 4 to 6 new INDs per year. This large variation stems from the large variability in willingness of companies to focus their research efforts early in the R&D process. Stepping back one step further into the exploratory research intended to identify potential drug development targets, we must again multiply the active drug development projects by a factor of 5 to 10. Therefore, one needs up to 1500 exploratory preclinical compounds at any given time to ultimately support filing of one approvable application per year (Table 1). Even in today's best case scenario, one needs 100 exploratory preclinical compounds to support one approvable application per year (Table 1). Table 1 summarizes these permutations. Clearly, focusing on 5 to 10 preclinical project areas presents a very different risk of failure to the corporation and requires very different resources than embracing 20 to 30 preclinical project areas and fostering equity-building collaborations to even further increase the probability of success.

This view paints a somewhat pessimistic picture of the probability of maintaining a record of success in clinical drug development. However, there are multiplicative beneficial outcomes from each successful drug development project. Success in a given research project is not likely to be an isolated success. Corporations who have spent the time and money to develop and retain research equity in a given area of drug development are more likely to succeed with follow-up compounds, line extensions, and even compounds in related areas as a result of their initial success. For example, each of us can name the pharmaceutical company most recognized for multiple successes in developing non-steroidal anti-inflammatory drugs, the company most recognized as a pioneer in commercial applications of biotechnology, and the company most known for multiple developments in the arena of controlled release of drugs. In order for subsequent related compounds to be developed expeditiously and efficiently, a corporation must retain the research equity gained from the initial successful project. Therein lies the importance of critical mass research teams. Their repetitive success in a single area of research offers an opportunity for the corporation to sustain strength, not only in that area, but even more importantly use their strength in one therapeutic area to acquire capabilities, technology, and other compounds. Such acquisitions may be of commercial value not only to the original therapeutic area, but to other areas that will benefit from transferable research equity.

Table 1. Permutations of various odds of sustaining a record of filing one approvable NDA per year.

	Stage of Drug Development Process					
	Exploratory Research Compound to	Preclinical Project Status to	IND Filed to	NDA Filed to	Approved New Chemical Entity	Overall Frequency of Compounds Resulting in an Approved NDA
Odds of Success at each Transition:						
"Best Case"	1/5	1/5	1/4	1		= 1/100
Other Case	1/10	1/25	1/6	1		= 1/1500

V. ESTABLISHING A CONTEXT FOR PRODUCT LICENSURE

In-licensing and out-licensing activities of the corporation are two tools that research management can use to integrate products from its own corporate research program into a stream of products for the income-generating side of the organization. Research management has the best opportunity to identify and understand the strengths and weaknesses of their overall research organization. Even in a widely recognized research organization such as Merck Sharp & Dohme, not all research endeavors succeed, and systems have been devised to assure that the good ideas are not lost in the process [9]. Few other organizations can boast the breadth and depth that characterize the Merck research operation. Moreover, the costly nature of drug development in today's world may preclude other organizations from developing resources similar to those at Merck. Indeed, the trend of most pharmaceutical research corporations is to focus on fewer therapeutic categories [10]. One can argue that this trend is increasing the cost of each discovery. However, that topic is not the focus of this chapter.

This chapter focuses on the realities of the research-marketing interface. One reality is that if individual organizations are going to focus more narrowly in their research endeavors, then it becomes an absolute necessity for them to optimize the income-generating potential of their successful drug development programs. Consequently, out-licensing follow-up compounds to generate royalty income or pursing them internally to approval becomes an absolute necessity resulting from the reduced opportunity that the research organization embraces by focusing their research on fewer targets. Further, focusing the intracompany research effort does not mean that a company's income-generating capabilities should be limited to the sale of products developed by its own well-targeted research. In-licensure of compounds may enable the marketing arm of the organization to exploit marketing capabilities and strengths in areas where the corporation has either not developed its research capabilities or has initiated a research program only in the recent past. Morgan [11] noted that business acquisitions are often pursued because they can be integrated to accomplish some strategic objective for the company's core activities. An in-licensing function may also enable the research organization to obtain complementary or synergistic technologies in new areas of research and thereby accelerate drug development via purchase of research equity. Such technological acquisition can be much faster than the slower process of growing all research equity internally. All of us recognize that it takes 10 years for a virgin research team to accumulate 10 years of experience! Table 2 summarizes the desirable features of in-licensed technologies.

Speed and flexibility have been touted as important qualities of any successful company today [12]. Changes in research direction may result

Table 2.   Desirable features of in-license technologies.

1. non-overlapping and complementary to existing products (e.g., acquisition of an oral quinolone antibiotic by a company marketing only parenteral antibiotics)
2. contribution to existing research equity (e.g., acquisition of a compound for inflammatory bowel disease by a company with active research on GI motility disorders)
3. potential for research synergy (e.g., acquisition of a selective leukotriene antagonist by a company already pursuing methylxanthines for asthma)
4. no competition for committed resources (e.g., it is not preferable to license a "me too" beta-blocker into a company already developing a novel antihypertensive drug)
5. no known data that is likely to impede approval of the drug candidate

in a corporation possessing research technologies that it does not wish to utilize. Changes may also put the company in the position to reconsider in-licensure of technologies that are no longer complementary to existing capabilities of the organization. Unless research management is willing to expand research capabilities to take advantage of and fully develop research equity in the area of acquired technology, such technologies may actually have a negative impact on both the research organization and the corporation's capacity to produce income. The reason for this negative impact is that the effort to develop and market a single compound in a new and unfamiliar therapeutic area is expensive, both in terms of direct costs and opportunity cost for the research and marketing arms of the organization. If these capabilities are used only once, then the corporation has only a single opportunity for return on investment. Consequently, the return must be very high to justify such an endeavor. Marketing considerations alone may lead to use of a lower threshold of return necessary to initiate such one-time projects. This approach fails to consider the very high opportunity cost of research equity that is not re-invested in another project.

This requirement for extraordinary return on investment is responsible for the increased risk that one must embrace in any isolated in-licensure activity. Despite the best efforts of a company to obtain the maximum amount of information about a licensure candidate, evaluations of in-licensure candidates will be based on less data than would be available for the evaluation of internal projects and technologies. Therein lies the major reason for all licensure activity (both in-licensure and out-licensure) to be part of the R&D operation. Evaluation of data on an acquisition candidate is most effectively performed by members of the R&D organization. In addition, R&D management must also evaluate the status of a given acquisition relative to other ongoing research projects. In the same context,

R&D management should be responsible for products that are being out-licensed in order to assure that the information required by the potential licensor for efficient evaluation is provided.

R&D management is in the best position to evaluate the necessity and utility of technologies for acquisition when the marketing side of the organization identifies a need with a specific window of opportunity. R&D management has the best opportunity to identify the most efficient approach to fitting in that window of opportunity. If R&D management has a number of intracompany products that appear to have appropriate timeframes of success, then in-licensure candidates can be evaluated to determine if they have a better market potential than the in-house product. In addition, the critical mass research teams must make recommendations on the likely impact of the acquisition on the research status of their programs. Sometimes, an in-licensure candidate may fit the window of opportunity better. If the marketing potential for such a product is adequate, in-licensure should proceed. In such endeavors, a cooperative approach between R&D and Marketing is vital to the overall success of the corporation.

REFERENCES

1. Peters T, Waterman RH. *In Search of Excellence*. New York: Harper & Row, Publishers, 1982.
2. Koberstein W. Executive profile: David Bethune. *Pharmaceutical Executive*, pp. 24–32, August, 1989.
3. Reidenberg MM. The state of drug development in the United States in 1990: a view from the academic community. *Clin. Pharmacol. Therap. 48*: 1–9 (1990).
4. Alzheimer A. A characteristic disease of the cerebral cortex. In: *The Early Story of Alzheimer's Disease* (Bick K, Amaducci L, Pepeu G, eds.). New York: Raven Press, pp. 1–3, 1987.
5. Wisniewski HM. Milestones in the history of Alzheimer disease research. In: *Alzheimer's Disease and Related Disorders* (Iqbal K, Wisniewski HM, Winblad B, eds.). New York: Alan R. Liss, Inc., pp. 1–11, 1989.
6. Padgett Lea P. Industry shooting stars blind Wall Street to long-term prospects. *Pharmaceutical Executive*, pp. 78–79, May, 1989.
7. Gupta AK, Wilemon D. Why R&D resists using marketing information. *Research Technology Management*, pp. 36–41, November–December, 1988.
8. Deshpande R, Zaltman G. Factors affecting the use of market research information: a path analysis. *Journal of Marketing Research 19*: 14–31 (February, 1982).
9. Weber J. A culture that keeps dishing up success. R&D muscle has brought Merck a steady-stream of top-selling drugs. *Business Week (Innovation in America)*, p. 120 (August, 1989).

10. Riccardo JP, Ryan BA. Pharmaceutical prospects in the post-lean and mean era. *Pharmaceutical Executive*, pp. 68–71, July, 1988.
11. Morgan G. *Riding the Waves of Change: Developing Managerial Competencies for a Turbulent World*. San Francisco: Jossey-Bass Publishers, pp. 131–132, 1988.
12. Dumaine B. How managers can succeed through speed. *Fortune* 119: 54–59 (February 13, 1989).

part four

The Past, the Present, and the Future of Clinical Drug Development

11

The Past: Major Laws Governing Clinical Drug Development in the United States

> The only thing new in the world
> is the history you don't know.
>
> *Harry S Truman*

I. INTRODUCTION

The purpose of this chapter is to provide general definition of the legal and regulatory environment within which clinical scientists work. We emphasize the historical milestones of drug law and indicate throughout this chapter that the arena of clinical drug development has become a pervasively regulated arena.

II. THE BEGINNINGS OF PHARMACEUTICAL LAW

Law often becomes a necessary control mechanism when people could be exploited and there are large potential financial gains for businesses choosing to exploit. For pharmaceuticals, the possibility of large financial gains emerged with the availability of patent protection in the late 1700s. The Patent Act of 1790 established market protection for certain medicines in the U.S. This Act established the period of protected exclusivity at 14 years, apparently since 14 years was equal to two periods of apprenticeship. Legislation in 1836 permitted the Commissioner of Patents to extend the 14 year period by an additional 7 years, but this extension was repealed in the Patent Act of 1861 which established the current seventeen-year patent term as a compromise between the original 14-year term and extended 21-year term. The 1861 Act established that a patentable invention must be (1) novel and not obvious and (2) a process, machine, manufacture, or composition of matter that is useful. Further, the 1861 Act established that the patent owner has the right to exclude others from making, using, or selling the invention in the U.S. Each patent includes specifications on how the invention is made, its uses, modes of application, and claims defining the boundaries of patent rights. Patent claims can cover a product (i.e., product patent), a process for product development (i.e., process patent), or a method for using the invention (i.e., use patent). Dr. Samuel Lee, an American physician in the 18th century, was the first holder of a U.S. patent for a drug or medical device.

In the late 1800s, quackery in medicines was widespread and it was reflected in extensive advertising in popular magazines such as *Harper's Weekly*. Young [1] noted that the 1876 volume of *Harper's Weekly* contained advertisements for products promising to cure asthma, cancer, cholera, consumption, diabetes, diphtheria, dyspepsia, epilepsy, gout, malaria, opium addiction, rheumatism, sea sickness, and yellow fever. These medicines included Kick-A-Poo Sagwa, Warner's Safe Diabetes Remedy, Mrs. Winslow's Soothing Syrup, Dr. Johnson's Mild Combination Treatment for Cancer, and Dr. Shreve's Anti-gall-stone Remedy. At that time, Listerine was sold to cure gonorrhea [1]. In view of the unregulated nature of such therapeutic claims, it is understandable that in 1900 patent medicines comprised the top category of spending for national advertising [1].

In viewing the need for early drug legislation, it is important to recall the nature of health care, especially drug therapy, in the late 1800s and early 1900s. Few effective drugs were available. Thomas [2] commented on this topic from his recollections of the state of medicine in the early 1900s. The year 1932 is often cited as the beginning of the modern era of drug discovery and development since it was the year that prontosil was developed. Scientists at the Pasteur Institute later discovered that sulfanilamide was the antibacterial moiety in the prontosil molecule. In the 1930s, patients with early stages of syphilis could be treated with arsphenamine. Morphine had proven value as an analgesic and digitalis had demonstrable benefit in some patients with cardiovascular disease. Pernicious anemia was treated successfully with liver extract (containing vitamin B12). Diptheria was amenable to treatment with antitoxin and prevention via immunization. Clearly, only a few therapies were available to treat a very limited number of diseases.

III. PHARMACOPOEIAS AS A MEANS TO SET STANDARDS FOR DRUG PRODUCTS

Standards of quality for drugs were not specified by any regulatory, scientific, or medical authority in the 1700s and early 1800s in the United States. This lack of legal and professional standards for drugs made the United States a dumping ground for the substandard and contaminated drugs that could not meet the legal and regulatory standards of European countries. In the early 1800s, physician sentiment moved toward creation of a pharmacopoeia as a means of increasing confidence in medicines. In 1817, Dr. Lyman Spalding submitted to the Medical Society of the County of New York a plan to create a national pharmacopoeia. The pharmacopoeia would be a compilation of specifications for drugs designed to bring about uniformity of composition, strength, and purity. The first *U.S. Pharmacopoeia* was published in December 1820 as a list of materia medica and a formulary of compositions to be made by the apothecary. It was sponsored by the collective authority of medical institutions whose representatives convened every 10 years. National pharmacist organizations did not exist at that time, but pharmacist cooperation was essential to success of the *U.S.P.*

The American Pharmaceutical Association was formed in 1852. The *National Formulary of Unofficial Preparations* was first issued in 1888 after being prepared and published by the national professional society of pharmacists.

The *American Homeopathic Pharmacopoeia* was first published in 1882 by the American Institute of Homeopathy. Later revisions to this book resulted in *The Homeopathic Pharmacopoeia of the United States* which became the sole authority for homeopathic remedies in the United States after recognition in the 1938 FD&C Act. One author speculated that this pharmacopoeia achieved legislative recognition because the sponsor of the bill in the Senate (Senator Royall S. Copeland, NY) was a homeopathic physician [3].

IV. EARLY FEDERAL LEGISLATION

The historical milestones of drug law are summarized in Table 1. The first attempt by the U.S. federal government to regulate the quality of drugs was passed in 1848 (Import Drugs Act). Earlier laws by individual states preceding enactment of this law have been discussed by Janssen [4,5]. The Import Drugs Act provided for laboratory inspection of imported drugs at the ports of entry in an effort to stop importation of impure and

Table 1. List of major legislation, regulations, and other milestones affecting
drug development and marketing in the United States.

1790	Patent Act
1819	Vaccine Law
1820	first U.S.P.
1848	Import Drugs Act
1861	Patent Act
1888	first National Formulary of Unofficial Preparations
1902	Biologics Control Act
1906	Pure Food and Drugs Act
1912	Sherley Amendment to Pure Food & Drugs Act
1914	Harrison Narcotic Act
1938	Federal Food, Drug and Cosmetic Act
1948	Miller Amendment
1951	Durham-Humphrey Amendments
1962	Drug (Kefauver-Harris) Amendments
1963	Initial Good Manufacturing Practices (GMPs) Regulations
1965	Drug Abuse Control Amendments
1968	Radiation Control for Health and Safety Act
1970	Poison Prevention Packaging Act
1970	Comprehensive Drug Abuse Prevention and Control Act
1972	Drug Listing Act
1976	Medical Device Act
1977	Proposed Establishment of Regulations on Obligations of Sponsors and Monitors
1978	Proposed Establishment of Regulations on Obligations of Clinical Investigators of Regulated Articles
1979	Drug Regulation Reform Act
1981	Final Rule/Regulations on Protection of Human Subjects/Informed Consent/Standards for Institutional Review Boards for Clinical Investigations; and Clinical Investigations Which May Be Reviewed Through Expedited Review Procedures
1983	Orphan Drug Act
1984	Drug Price Competition and Patent Term Restoration Act
1985	NDA Rewrites
1987	IND Rewrites
1987	Treatment IND regulations
1987	Prescription Drug Marketing Act
1988	Subpart E regulations

contaminated drug products. Further, such unacceptable products could be re-exported or retained for destruction. This Act was meant to stop importation of adulterated quinine for sale to American troops who were fighting in the Spanish-American war. Much was yet to come as an 1849 editorial stated that the Act was a first step in ". . . necessary reforms of a monstrous evil" [6].

A long series of distinguished individuals led the Bureau of Chemistry and FDA (Table 2). In 1883, Dr. Harvey Washington Wiley was appointed Chief Chemist of the U. S. Department of Agriculture. His predecessor, Peter Collier, had supported earlier unsuccessful efforts to pass a federal law prohibiting adulteration of food. However, it remained for Dr. Wiley to invest the better part of his career in achieving passage of such legislation.

Dr. Wiley was trained as a chemist and physician. Most of his effort was directed towards exploring the concept that food additives and preservatives should be used in a concentration range allowing for an adequate separation between effective use of these agents and any hazardous effects of these agents. The increasing urbanization and industrialization at the turn of the century led to a need to process, store, and ship foods. Dr. Wiley was concerned about the use of certain food preservatives (e.g., formaldehyde, borax) and food additives (e.g., copper sulfate to enhance the green color of vegetables). In order to study the properties of food additives and preservatives in man, Dr. Wiley formed the "poison squad." This poison squad consisted of a group of healthy, adult, male volunteers who received controlled diets containing experimental additives. Experimentation with the poison squad began on December 16, 1902 and continued for several years. Many purported preservatives, including boric acid, borax, formaldehyde, potassium nitrate, salicylates, and sulfurous acid, were evaluated [7,8]. Although not initiated for publicity, these "poison squad" experiments were the basis of considerable publicity for Dr. Wiley's efforts toward legislation. Of course, Dr. Wiley served as Chief Chemist during an era, i.e., the late 1800's, when freedom of action with minimal governmental regulation was the predominant pattern of social action in the United States. Therefore, he founded a long and arduous effort to move towards legislation governing the safe use of food additives. More than 100 bills proposing food or drug legislation were introduced into Congress from 1879 to 1906, but tragic events were essential to precipitate legislative action.

The nation's first regulatory program for biologics was enacted in 1902 as the Biologics Control Act. This Act gave the U.S. Public Health Service the control over licensing of biologics laboratories and their products. Passage of the Act was precipitated in 1902 by the death of 12 children

Table 2. Listing of historical directors of the Department of Agriculture, Bureau of Chemistry, and Food and Drug Administration.

Name and Title	Term of Office	Concurrent Presidential Terms
Charles M. Wetherill Chemist, U.S. Dept. of Agriculture	1862–1863	Abraham Lincoln
Henri Erni Chemist, U.S. Dept. of Agriculture	1863–1866	Abraham Lincoln Andrew Johnson
Thomas Antisell, M.D. Chemist, U.S. Dept. of Agriculture	1867–1870	Andrew Johnson Ulysses S. Grant
Ryland T. Brown Chemist, U.S. Dept. of Agriculture	1871–1873	Ulysses S. Grant
William McMurtie Chemist, U.S. Dept. of Agriculture	1874–1878	Ulysses S. Grant Rutherford B. Hayes
Peter Collier Chemist, U.S. Dept. of Agriculture	1879–1883	Rutherford B. Hayes James A. Garfield Chester A. Arthur
Harvey W. Wiley, M.D. Chief, Bureau of Chemistry U.S. Dept. of Agriculture	1883–1912	Chester A. Arthur Grover Cleveland Benjamin Harrison William McKinley Theodore Roosevelt William H. Taft
Carl L. Alsberg, M.D. Chief, Bureau of Chemistry U.S. Dept. of Agriculture	1912–1921	William H. Taft Woodrow Wilson
Walter G. Campbell Acting Chief, Bureau of Chemistry, U.S. Dept. of Agriculture	1921–1923	Warren G. Harding
Charles A. Browne, Ph.D. Chief, Bureau of Chemistry U.S. Dept. of Agriculture	1923–1927	Calvin Coolidge
Walter G. Campbell Directory of Regulatory Work, U.S.D.A.	1927–1940	Calvin Coolidge Herbert Hoover Franklin D. Roosevelt
Commissioner of Food & Drugs, U.S.D.A.	1940–1944	
Paul B. Dunbar, Ph.D. Commissioner of Food & Drugs Federal Security Agency	1944–1951	Franklin D. Roosevelt Harry S Truman

Table 2   (*Continued*)

Name and Title	Term of Office	Concurrent Presidential Terms
Charles W. Crawford Commissioner of Food & Drugs Food & Drug Administration	1951–1954	Harry S Truman Dwight D. Eisenhower
George P. Larrick Commissioner of Food & Drugs FDA, Dept. of HEW	1954–1965	Dwight D. Eisenhower John F. Kennedy Lyndon B. Johnson
James L. Goddard, MD, MPH Commissioner of Food & Drugs FDA, Dept. of HEW	1966–1968	Lyndon B. Johnson
Herbert L. Ley, Jr., MD, MPH Commissioner of Food & Drugs FDA, Dept. of HEW	1968–1969	Lyndon B. Johnson
Charles C. Edwards, M.D. Commissioner of Food & Drugs FDA, Dept. of HEW	1969–1973	Richard M. Nixon
Alexander M. Schmidt, M.D. Commissioner of Food & Drugs FDA, Dept. of HEW	1973–1976	Richard M. Nixon Gerald R. Ford
Donald Kennedy, Ph.D. Commissioner of Food & Drugs FDA, Dept. of HEW	1977–1979	Jimmy Carter
Jere E. Goyan, Ph.D. Commissioner of Food & Drugs FDA, Dept. of HEW	1979–1981	Jimmy Carter
Arthur Hull Hayes, Jr., M.D. Commissioner of Food & Drugs FDA, Dept. of HHS	1981–1983	Ronald Reagan
Frank E. Young, M.D., Ph.D. Commissioner of Food & Drugs FDA, Dept. of HHS	1984–1989	Ronald Reagan George Bush
David A. Kessler, MD, JD Commissioner of Food & Drugs FDA, Dept. of HHS	1990–present	George Bush

from tetanus contamination of a diphtheria antitoxin made by the St. Louis Health Department [4,9].

After passage of the 1902 Act, Dr. Wiley continued to lead the crusade for further federal legislation with his grassroots speaking program at civic and women's clubs. Muckraking journalists supported the campaign with articles in high circulation magazines of the time, such as *Collier's Weekly*, *Ladies Home Journal*, and *Good Housekeeping*. A classic article entitled "The Great American Fraud" by Samuel Hopkins Adams appeared in *Collier's* in 1905. A copy of this vibrant article was graciously provided to the authors by the FDA Historian (Mr. Wallace F. Janssen) and we are happy to provide a copy to interested parties.

Opposition to further legislation came principally from the many manufacturers of patent medicines and distillers. These companies feared the potentially catastrophic effects of legislation and regulation on their businesses. Twenty-three years after the appointment of Dr. Wiley, the Federal Pure Food and Drugs Act was passed on June 30, 1906 following signature by President Theodore Roosevelt. The Federal Pure Food and Drugs Act required that drugs marketed in commerce meet their stated minimum standards of strength, purity, and quality, i.e., no product could be adulterated (i.e., impure). This act also recognized for the first time the *National Formulary* and *United States Pharmacopoeia* as the official compendia acceptable within the United States. *The Homeopathic Pharmacopoeia of the United States* was later added as a recognized pharmacopoeia in 1938. The 1906 Act was signed into law only after a serious precipitating event. Enactment of the 1906 law followed twenty-three years of work by Dr. Wiley's group, support by organized medical societies, and support by the press and organized women's groups, but was precipitated by revelations in Adams' article in 1905 and disclosures of the unsanitary conditions in the meat packing industry in Chicago as described in the book *The Jungle* by Upton Sinclair [10].

The 1906 Pure Food and Drugs Act did suffer a number of major deficiencies. Most notably, the law provided no provision for assessment of the safety or efficacy of drugs. Further, the law did not regulate the labeling and therapeutic claims made for products by pharmaceutical manufacturers. Also, the law did not extend to cosmetics. Finally, the law required labeling of only the quantity of certain substances (e.g., ethanol, morphine, opium, heroin, cocaine, chloroform, cannabis, and chloral hydrate) without restriction on their therapeutic claims. This allowed, for example, continued promotion and sale of morphine-containing soothing syrups for relief of teething discomfort in infants! Penalties for violation of the Act were mild. With the support of President Taft, the Sherley Amendment was passed to the Pure Food and Drugs Act in 1912. President William Howard Taft urged passage of this amendment with the statement [4]:

There are none so credulous as sufferers from disease. The need is urgent for legislation that will prevent the raising the false hopes of speedy cures of serious ailments by misstatements of facts as to worthless mixtures on which the sick will rely while their disease progresses unchecked.

The Sherley Amendment was the first federal legislation to regulate labeling. This amendment was the legislative introduction of the term "misbranded" as it referred to fraudulent or false claims of therapeutic effects. However, a violation of this law could only be established if the plaintiff could prove that the seller intended to deliberately defraud the buyer. The necessity to prove intent to defraud made the Sherley Amendment a weak improvement to the original 1906 Act.

In 1927, enforcement of the Pure Food and Drugs Act was moved from the Bureau of Chemistry to the Food, Drug, and Insecticide Administration within the Department of Agriculture. In 1931, reorganization in the federal government led to formation of the Food and Drug Administration as a separate agency within the U.S. Department of Agriculture. Later in 1940, FDA was transferred to the Federal Security Agency, i.e., the predecessor of the Department of Health, Education, and Welfare, now known as the Department of Health and Human Services.

V. FEDERAL FOOD, DRUG AND COSMETIC ACT

Events in the late 1930s followed the pattern in 1905 and 1906 whereby a precipitating medical-social event led to passage of major legislation governing marketing and development of drugs in the United States. In 1937, a U.S. health crisis occurred from the use of elixir sulfanilamide, a new antibacterial product. Sulfanilamide was one of an initial family of sulfa antibiotics that had broad utility in a variety of patient populations with a variety of bacterial infectious diseases. Sulfanilamide was marketed initially in tablet dosage forms which had limited usefulness for treatment of pediatric patients. The S.E. Massengill Company had a particular interest in developing a formulation of sulfanilamide to provide a good tasting, liquid product for treatment of children with streptococcal pharyngitis. The Massengill Company's chief chemist and pharmacist (Harold Cole Watkins) succeeded in formulating a sweet, raspberry-flavored liquid which was deemed acceptable after testing in the laboratory for flavor, aroma, and appearance. No animal or human studies were conducted on this product prior to marketing [11,12]. The elixir sulfanilamide was introduced to the U.S. market on September 4, 1937. Shortly thereafter, reports of deaths of pediatric and adult patients began to emerge. The initial fatality report was received on October 14, 1937; it was not reported to Food and Drug Administration, but rather to the American Medical Association by a physician in Tulsa, Oklahoma. Ultimately, a total of 107 patients were known fatalities [7]. Patients died of acute renal failure. This product was later learned to contain diethylene glycol; the presence of this compound comprised its misbranding as an elixir which enabled Food and Drug Administration to seize the product as ordered on October 16, 1937; FDA recovered 99.2% of the product in distribution [13]. Of the 240 gallons manufactured and distributed by Massengill Co., 234 gallons and 1 pint were retrieved by FDA [12]. Ethylene glycol is now known to be metabolized in man to the nephrotoxin, oxalic acid. Ethylene glycol is well known today for its use in automotive antifreeze. It is noteworthy that FDA was not able to seize this product on the grounds that it was unsafe for human use or adulterated. Conceivably, labeling this product as a solution would have rendered it within the law. Marketing of elixir sulfanilamide proved to be a devastating occurrence in the history of drug safety regulation and pediatric care, as well as a devastating occurrence for the chemist who developed this formulation since he committed suicide after being informed of the product-related fatalities.

The elixir sulfanilamide disaster led in 1938 to passage of the Federal Food, Drug and Cosmetic Act. The FD&C Act extended the prior Pure Food and Drugs Act of 1906 in several major ways. The FD&C Act required predistribution clearance for safety of new drugs, thereby representing the first legislative act which necessitated demonstration of safety prior to approval for marketing. The FD&C Act also extended coverage from foods and drugs to cosmetics and medical devices. The Act expanded the meaning of adulteration and misbranding by requiring that labels ("displays of written, printed, or graphic matter upon the immediate container of any article") provide adequate directions for use to the consumer. Drugs containing certain narcotic or hypnotic ingredients were required to state on the label "Warning: May be habit forming." Finally, the Act served to authorize representatives of FDA to inspect the factories of pharmaceutical manufacturers.

VI.   AMENDMENTS TO THE FD&C ACT

A.   Batch Certification of Insulin and Penicillin

In 1941, the FD&C Act was amended to require batch certification of the safety and activity of insulin. Insulin was the first biologically derived hormone to require certification of activity prior to market introduction. The FD&C Act was further amended in 1945 to require certification of safety and activity of penicillin batches. These provisions for batch certification were later extended in 1962 to all antibiotics intended for use in man.

B. Miller Amendment and Durham-Humphrey Amendment

Regulations governing drug labeling were amended in 1945 to clarify the distinction between prescription drugs and non-prescription drugs. These regulations required that (1) drugs commonly purchased and suitable for use by lay consumers without the intervention of professional guidance must bear adequate directions for use, (2) drugs dangerous for use without the supervision of a physician are exempted from the need to be labeled with directions for use since presence of such directions may encourage self-medication, and (3) drugs requiring medical skill for proper use (e.g., certain injectables) are exempt from the need to be labeled with directions for use. Interestingly, these regulations required manufacturers to omit directions for use and indications from the labeling of packages of prescription drugs, thereby preserving the situation where only the physician and not the patient knew the identity of the medicine. Note that these 1945 instruments of change were regulations and there was still no law defining prescription versus non-prescription drugs.

The legal basis for discerning prescription versus non-prescription drugs was established in 1951 with a major amendment to the FD&C Act. At that time, the Durham-Humphrey amendment was introduced in order to define these two separate classes of drug products. The need for this statutory definition of prescription drug was heightened in 1948. In that year, the Supreme Court ruled in the Sullivan case that a pharmacist who sold sulfathiazole without a prescription violated the misbranding provision of the FD&C Act by not providing the patient with adequate directions for use and adequate warnings [14]. Subsequently, pharmacists began to express further concern about the need for a statutory definition of prescription drug when the 1948 Miller Amendment to the FD&C Act extended the applicability of the Act to wholesale and retail providers of drugs, in addition to the previous coverage of manufacturers. This amendment, together with the earlier ruling in the Sullivan case, heightened concern by retail pharmacists that they could be prosecuted for selling legend drugs without a prescription. At that time, the same chemical drug was labeled by some manufacturers with adequate directions for use, while other manufacturers labeled the same drug with the Rx legend ("Caution: to be used only by or on prescription of a physician."). Under the Miller

Amendment and in accordance with the precedent ruling in the Sullivan case, a pharmacist would be in violation of the FD&C Act if he dispensed a legend drug (i.e., a drug without adequate directions for use in the labeling) to a patient without a prescription. To remove this liability, a clarifying amendment to the FD&C Act was needed.

Major support for the Durham-Humphrey Amendment came from FDA and the National Association of Retail Druggists. Through the Durham-Humphrey Amendment, prescription drugs were defined as (1) hypnotic or habit forming drugs (and their derivatives) that are specifically named in the law, (2) a drug unsafe for self-medication because of its toxicity or other potentiality for harmful effect or the method of its use or the collateral measures necessary to its use, or (3) a new drug not shown to be safe for use in self-medication. One practical consequence of the Durham-Humphrey Amendment for the pharmacist was creation of a class of drugs exempt from the requirement that their labels provide adequate directions for use. This class of drugs was deemed safe for use only under medical supervision and they were required to bear the legend. These legend drugs were exempt from labeling provisions if they were administered under a prescriber's supervision or sold pursuant to the order of a licensed prescriber. The amendment also introduced the requirement for addition of the prescription legend on the label of all U.S. prescriptions delivered to patients. This legend states "Caution: Federal law prohibits dispensing without a prescription." Further, refills of a prescription were prohibited except on authorization from the prescriber.

The regulations governing labeling were the next major component to be overhauled. As a result of the Durham-Humphrey Amendment, prescription drugs did not come in bottles containing information or directions for use. This "information deficit" was consistent with the common notion that only the prescribing physician and not the patient should have access to such information. However, the changing sentiment at the time is captured in this statement from Dr. Ralph G. Smith, then Director of FDA's Division of New Drugs [4]:

> The drug manufacturers were replacing the medical schools as the principal source of information for physicians in their use of new drugs. The informative labeling worked out by FDA with applicants in the course of processing New Drug Applications, was not reaching physicians. This labeling, in accord with the regulations, was referred to on the drug label as "available to physicians on request." The pharmaceutical industry, however, was promoting the use of these potent new drugs to physicians by detail men, mailing pieces, medical journal advertising, and reference publi-

cations that frequently failed to disclose their hazards. The more informative labeling was usually not part of the drug package and was rarely requested by the physician, nor was there any assurance it would be included in a response to a request for information. As the dangers of this situation were recognized, FDA's division of new drugs increasingly required the informative labeling to be made a part of the prescription drug package. This was not an adequate solution to the problem and in 1961 the so-called "full disclosure" regulations were promulgated.

Therefore, proposed regulations published in the *Federal Register* on July 22, 1960 called for inclusion of complete professional information (i.e., a "package insert") in virtually all packages of prescription drugs and promotional literature. Final regulations were issued on December 9, 1960. The proposal to make the package insert the vehicle of professional information was issued in regulations of September 6, 1961 under FDA Commissioner Larrick, despite opposition from the American Medical Association [15].

C. Kefauver-Harris Amendments

Further major amendments to the FD&C act were introduced in 1962. The Drug Amendments of 1962 (Kefauver-Harris amendments) established for the first time that proof of efficacy was required prior to marketing a drug. This legislation followed Senate hearings conducted in the late 1950s and early 1960s. These hearings were chaired by Tennessee Senator Estes Kefauver on issues of marketing and pricing of drug products. The senate subcommittee was motivated by (1) drug prices that were considered high and monopolistically noncompetitive, (2) lack of demonstrated efficacy of existing and new drugs, (3) minimal reporting by drug companies to doctors and regulators of adverse effects of drugs, and (4) lack of effective means to track and recall dangerous investigational drugs.

Senator Kefauver's original bill was targeted to promote increased industrial competition and thereby lower drug prices. The counterpart bill within the House of Representatives was sponsored by Representative Orrin Harris (Arkansas), chairman of the House Committee on Interstate and Foreign Commerce. The original bills seemed unlikely to pass. However, the Senate bill was modified to incorporate items from another bill (M.R. 1235; originally proposed by Missouri Representative Leonor K. Sullivan). Representative Sullivan was the first member of Congress to propose that efficacy requirements be introduced in federal drug legislation.

The precipitating factor that spurred passage of the amendments was the tragedy of thalidomide-related phocomelia reported in late 1961 in the

U.K., Sweden, Italy, Scotland, Switzerland, Lebanon, Israel, Australia, Brazil, Peru, and West Germany. Thalidomide was a sedative-hypnotic agent developed by the West German company Chemie Grunenthal. It had utility in facilitating rest in pregnant women, as well as other patients. Thalidomide was marketed in several European countries for about three years before reports appeared of the association between thalidomide and phocomelia [11]. Chemie Grunenthal withdrew all forms of thalidomide from distribution and sale in November, 1961. Merrell withdrew the drug in Canada in February, 1962.

Thalidomide was never approved for use in the U.S. Despite licensure of the product to the William S. Merrell Co., conduct of clinical investigations in the U.S, and filing an application for marketing, approval was never granted by FDA. Lack of approval was due to the absence of sufficient safety data (as required by the 1938 FD&C Act) to convince the medical officer (Frances O. Kelsey, M.D., Ph.D.) of the product's safety [11]. Dr. Kelsey's concern arose from reports in the British Medical Journal [16,17] suggesting that certain neuropathies may be related to thalidomide. She was aware from her laboratory research that drugs that caused neuropathies in adult rabbits could stunt growth and produce deformity in rabbit fetuses. In the U.S., Merrell had sent supplies of this investigational drug to approximately 1200 doctors [18]. Estimates were that 20,000 patients had received the drug in the U.S. [18]. A survey conducted by FDA showed that thalidomide had been given in the United States to 3,879 women of childbearing age and 9 of these women gave birth to infants with phocomelia [13]. Merrell was required only to keep a record of shipping and to label the drug for investigational use. Physician recipients were required to sign a statement that they were qualified to test the drug. Physicians were not required to inform their patients that the drug was investigational.

The thalidomide story demonstrated the presence of the following flaws in federal drug legislation: (1) no efficient means was in place to recall dangerous investigational drugs, (2) dissemination of investigational drugs to physicians was poorly controlled, (3) there was no means to assure that patients knew of the investigational nature of the drug prior to their decision to receive it as treatment, and (4) no assurance that physicians maintained adequate records regarding either the patients who received the drug or the effects that these patients experienced.

Until 1963, the drug review process in FDA did not begin until a *completed* NDA was filed. The sponsor was required to keep on file for 3 years the investigators statements of qualifications and physical equipment (if any) needed to conduct tasks. However, these items were unlikely to be scrutinized before NDA submission and did not have to be submitted in an IND. FDA took action before passage of the Kefauver-Harris Amendments. New regulations required drug sponsors to (1) inform FDA about distribution of drugs for investigational use, (2) collaborate only with qualified investigators whose qualifications were to be filed with the FDA, (3) test no new drugs in humans until reasonable limits of safety had been established in animals, (4) inform FDA of the progress of human testing, and (5) take special precautions with drugs intended for use by children or pregnant women. In addition, drug companies were required to register with FDA and undergo inspection at least once every 2 years, adverse events had to be reported to FDA, advertising of prescription drugs was required to provide fair balance of risks and benefits, and informed consent must be obtained from each patient prior to study. Perhaps most importantly, both safety and efficacy of a new drug was required to be demonstrated via substantial evidence prior to marketing. Pursuant to the Kefauver-Harris Amendment, Section 505(d) of Title 21 of the Code of Federal Regulations now requires that FDA reject any new drug application that lacks substantial evidence that the drug has the claimed effects and that this substantial evidence consist of adequate and well-controlled investigations, including clinical trials. Table 3 summarizes the characteristics of adequate and well controlled investigations as defined consistent with this legislation.

Table 3. Definition of adequate and well-controlled trial (abstracted from 21 CFR 314.126).

An "adequate and well-controlled study" has the following prospective characteristics:
1. clear statement of the objectives
2. description of the proposed methods of data analysis
3. the study design is described in full
4. the study design permits a valid comparison with an appropriate control
5. the study design provides a quantitative assessment of drug effect; variables to be measured must be specified with methodology for measurement
6. a statement whether sample size is preset by some method or to be based on interim analyses
7. subjects were selected in a manner to assure that they have the target disease
8. patients are assigned to treatments in a way that minimizes bias
9. measures are taken to minimize bias on the part of patients, investigators, and analysts of the data (e.g., blinding)
10. test drug must be standardized (for identity, strength, quality, purity, etc.)

The nature of substantial evidence of safety and efficacy has been the subject of debate. It is noteworthy that a precedent-setting legal case of Weinberger vs. Henson, Westcott, and Dunning was considered by the Supreme Court [19]. The Supreme Court rejected the use of testimonial evidence in constituting substantial evidence of support of a new drug application. The Supreme Court ruled "The substantial evidence requirement reflects the conclusion of Congress, based upon hearings, that clinical impressions of practicing physicians do not constitute an adequate basis for establishing efficacy."

The consequences of the Kefauver-Harris Amendments were, in some ways, staggering to the U.S. pharmaceutical industry. Prior to the Amendments, the manufacturer was obligated to produce an adequately labeled (i.e., not misbranded), appropriately constituted (i.e., not adulterated) product that was proven safe for human use. Passage of the Kefauver-Harris Amendments added the requirement that the sponsor produce substantial evidence of efficacy of the product for the stated claims; such substantial evidence must be collected in adequate and well-controlled investigations. This requirement for evidence of efficacy was further intensified by its retroactive application to all drugs approved between 1938 and 1962. The requirements of the Kefauver-Harris Amendment resulted in increased workload in the U.S. pharmaceutical industry and diminished effective patent life for new chemical entities.

The peak of approval of new drugs occurred in 1955 with 357 new drug applications receiving approval from FDA. Thereafter, there was a steady decline in approval of new applications. Interestingly, the number of NCEs approved and the number of NCEs offering important therapeutic gain has remained relatively constant since 1963 [20]. As indicated in Chapter 1, an average of 21.7 new chemical entities have been approved per year during the 1980s with 13% of these offering an important therapeutic advance.

VII. THE DESI PROJECT

Many drug products were approved as safe in accordance with the 1938 FD&C Act, but prior to passage of the 1962 Kefauver-Harris Amendments. The 1938 Act required these products to be cleared for safety; the 1962 Amendment required that the efficacy of these products be reviewed retrospectively while the product could remain on the market. Efficacy of these products was reviewed retrospectively via the Drug Efficacy Study Implementation Project (DESI). According to the 1962 Amendment, manufacturers were given 2 years after the date of effect of this law to provide FDA with substantial evidence of effectiveness for their claims. FDA contracted with the National Academy of Sciences/National Research Council on June 17, 1966 for conduct of the study known as the "Drug Efficacy Study of the Academy-Research Council." NAS/NRC assembled 30 panels of medical and scientific experts to assess the information available on drug products initially marketed between 1938 and 1962. NAS/NRC panels used information submitted by manufacturers, results published in the medical literature, and judgement to render their recommendations as reported to FDA in 1969 [21-23]. NAS/NRC recommended 16,537 effectiveness judgements for indications for the 3,443 drug products they evaluated [22]. Following these recommendations, the DESI project began its work. Although both prescription and non-prescription drugs were initially part of the DESI project, non-prescription drugs left DESI for evaluation under the OTC monograph procedures established in 1972. The DESI review started January 23, 1968. Approximately 7,700 drug products were removed from the market due to lack of substantial evidence of efficacy for all claims and an additional 3,500 drug products were removed from the market due to lack of applications on file with FDA [22]. Of the 3,443 drug products reviewed in the DESI Project, 3,232 drug products have received final action with 2,212 (68.5%) effective for all indications; 1,020 drug products (31.5%) lacking substantial evidence of efficacy; and 211 products still under review [22].

VIII. ANDA, PAPER NDA, AND OTHER MEANS FOR GENERIC PRODUCTS TO ENTER THE PHARMACEUTICAL MARKET

The history and regulatory evolution of the abbreviated NDA (ANDA), paper NDA, and Drug Price Competition and Patent Term Restoration Act (DPC-PTR) can only be fully appreciated by reviewing the chronological sequence of changes to the legal and regulatory barriers to the pharmaceutical market. Some excellent sources of extensive information already exist [24,25] and the major events will be summarized here.

The 1938 FD&C Act requires a potential manufacturer of any "new drug" to file an NDA and obtain approval for the NDA before initiating marketing. From 1938 through 1969, most generic drugs were marketed in the U.S. without filing or gaining approval for an NDA since these products claimed to be "not new drugs." A given generic drug claimed to be therapeutically equivalent to a pioneer product for which an approved NDA did exist. This situation changed dramatically in the late 1960s and early 1970s due to four major policy developments: (1) initiation in 1968 of clinical efficacy testing on currently marketed pioneer and generic drugs while marketing continued (i.e., the DESI review), (2) establishment in 1970 of the ANDA process as a means of premarketing clearance of generic drugs, (3) continuation in 1974 of protection of a pioneer's clinical safety and efficacy data as trade secrets or confidential commercial information under the Freedom of Information Act [26], and (4) implementation in 1978 of a "paper-NDA policy." We will expand on each of these four developments.

The Kefauver-Harris Amendments of 1962 required FDA to review the evidence of efficacy for each drug approved between 1938 and 1962. This review was executed as the DESI Project. The DESI review proceeded while pre-1962 drugs remained on the market. Further, the results of the DESI review were to categorize many drugs as possibly effective, thereby requiring new clinical studies to fully prove efficacy (so-called Paragraph XIV products). As long as the performance of new studies was diligently pursued, the drug could continue to be marketed. For drugs marketed by more than one company, it was not clear initially whether each company had to conduct its own clinical studies in order to continue marketing its own product. One notice from FDA suggested that studies done in collaboration by several manufacturers of one drug were an acceptable basis for all manufacturers to continue marketing [27]. Ultimately, the policy adopted by FDA stated that marketing may continue by all manufacturers as long as any one manufacturer is conducting the necessary new clinical studies [28]:

> In the interest of minimizing duplicative and costly clinical testing of essentially the same drug product, which places a burden on already overloaded and scarce clinical testing resources without necessarily contributing to the quality of evidence required to establish the drug's effectiveness, the Commissioner of Food and Drugs now concludes that each manufacturer need not clinically test its own product as long as at least one other manufacturer, or a consortium of manufacturers, is conducting tests on a product to which the same effectiveness conclusions would ultimately apply.

A. ANDAs and Paper NDAs

The ANDA (abbreviated NDA) process was established in 1970 as a means for premarketing clearance of generic drugs. An ANDA consists of information on manufacturing of the generic product, as well as scientific data demonstrating that the generic product is bioequivalent to the pioneer version of the product. An ANDA can be done for a generic equivalent to a pioneer drug originally approved prior to the 1962 Kefauver-Harris Amendment and found to be effective under the DESI project. An ANDA must contain a table of contents; label and all other labeling; a statement as to its intended use on a prescription basis or OTC; a full list of the articles used as components of the drug product; brief information on the drug product's composition and manufacture; and proof of bioequivalence. An ANDA is "abbreviated" in that nonclinical laboratory studies and clinical investigations are not conducted on the generic product. At the time of initiation of the ANDA process, FDA informed manufacturers of generic drugs of the requirement for an approved NDA for each generic product, including generic products already marketed and generic products not yet marketed [29]. For marketed products, FDA allowed marketing to continue if an ANDA was submitted for approval. Although some new generic products were allowed to enter the market at the time of submission of an ANDA, the final policy called for each new generic drug to attain approval for its ANDA before initiation of marketing [25].

The strength of the Freedom of Information Act (FOIA) was tested as a means of protecting the safety and efficacy data in the NDA for a pioneer drug. Availability of these data in the public domain would enable their use in NDAs for competitive generic products. In 1974, FOIA adhered to historical policy that such data were eligible for exemption from disclosure under FOIA due to their nature as trade secrets and confidential commercial information [26]. This decision favors exclusivity and hence innovation, rather than immediate marketing of generic drugs [30]:

> The public is dependent upon private pharmaceutical manufacturers for development of drugs. In some instances those drugs may be patented, but in other instances they may not be patented. If a manufacturer's safety and effectiveness data are to be released upon request, thus permitting "me-too" drugs to be marketed immediately, it is entirely possible that the incentive for private pharmaceutical research will be adversely affected.
>
> The Commissioner does not believe that this issue can or should be addressed by the Food and Drug Administration alone. Rather, it is an important public policy issue that can and should be addressed primarily by Congress.

This series of events in the late 1960s and early 1970s resulted in a series of actions by FDA to determine how new generic drugs would enter the market and how marketed generic drugs would stay on the market. Since the ANDA policy applied only to generic forms of pioneer drugs approved before 1962, great impending controversy was anticipated as the first post-1962 drugs approached the end of their patent lives. FDA estimated that about half of the top 200 prescription drugs in the U.S. would go off patent between 1977 and 1982 [25]. In 1974, FDA reported its inability to address this issue alone [30] and FDA (with Department of HEW) referred the matter to Congress. This referral resulted in a new proposed law, the Drug Regulation Reform Act of 1978. Although this legislation was never enacted, it proposed to provide a minimum 5-year marketing exclusivity period to each pioneer product. During this period, no generic products would be approved without the pioneer's consent. After this period and regardless of patent status, FDA would approve each generic product that met the requirements for identity, quality, and labeling. Issues of patent infringement would be contested by the pioneer company in court. Interestingly, in 1979, the Drug Regulation Improvement Act was proposed in the Senate. Although it contained the same exclusivity period to prohibit ANDAs for 5 years after approval of the pioneer NDA and it passed the Senate, it was never enacted.

Therefore, in 1978, FDA was facing a large number of post-1962 drugs that were beginning to go off patent, yet FDA still had no legislation to address the process by which generic equivalents of these drugs could seek an approved NDA. The so-called "paper-NDA policy" was implemented in 1978 in order to provide a means of approval of NDAs (under the Federal FD&C Act) based solely on published scientific papers in the absence of the underlying raw data, i.e., the case reports for each individual patient who participated in clinical research on the drug. FDA emphasized that the published reports must meet the criteria of adequate and well-controlled clinical trials in order to support approval of a paper NDA [31,32]. Paper NDAs were instituted by a policy memorandum issued by Dr. Marion J. Finkel, then Associate Director for New Drug Evaluation in FDA [31]. This policy was intended for use on an interim basis and it was intended only to be applied to those drugs approved after 1962.

Basically, FDA was looking for an "ANDA-like" policy to apply to generic equivalents of pioneer products that were approved after 1962. FDA continued to require a full NDA for any proposed generic form of a pioneer drug approved after 1962. This requirement was challenged by the first paper NDA as submitted by IMS Limited. This manufacturer submitted a paper NDA for a generic drug (furosemide) based on published reports on the safety and efficacy of the drug (in the absence of any original case reports) along with information on manufacturing and bioequivalency. During the period of review of this NDA, Dr. Finkel issued the policy memorandum. The relevant section states as follows [31]:

A drug marketed for the first time after 1962 under an approved new drug application may be marketed by a second firm only after the second firm has received the approval of a full new drug application for that product. Current agency policy does not permit ANDAs for this purpose. Present interpretation of the law is that no data in an NDA can be utilized to support another NDA without express permission of the original NDA holder. Thus, in the case of duplicate NDAs for already approved post-1962 drugs, the agency will accept published reports as the main supporting documentation for safety and effectiveness. The agency will not interpret the "full reports of investigations" phrase in the law [21 U.S.C. 355(b)(1)] as requiring either case reports or an exhaustive review of all published reports on the drug. Depending upon the quality of the published data, selected preclinical and perhaps additional clinical studies may be required of the new sponsor prior to NDA approval.

In accordance with this policy, the NDA submitted by IMS Limited was approved in January, 1979 as the first approval of a post-1962 drug entirely based on reports in the literature [25]. It is noteworthy that development and implementation of the paper-NDA policy began outside the usual channels of a proposed rule, public review of the proposed rule, then final implementation. The paper NDA policy was to be a temporary measure until the Drug Regulation Reform Act of 1978 was approved or until FDA brought post-1962 drugs into the DESI review or ANDA systems [31].

B. Drug Price Competition and Patent Term Restoration Act (Waxman-Hatch Amendments)

The Drug Price Competition and Patent Term Restoration Act of 1984 (DPC-PTR Act) was signed into law by President Reagan on September 24, 1984. It was the most important change in drug law since 1962. DPC-PTR Act provided the first means to extend a patent term since 1861 when the current 17 year patent was established. Title I of this Act amends the FD&C Act to establish provisions for approval by FDA of applications for generic versions of pioneer drugs approved at any time (i.e., pre-1962 or post-1962) under the FD&C Act. Title II amends the patent laws to provide for restoration of part of the patent term which was used for the clinical testing period and the FDA review period for a new drug. It also awards an exclusivity period for significant new findings about a previously approved drug. Title III of the Act is unrelated to patent term restoration or ANDAs and it is not discussed here.

1. History of DPC-PTR Act

The 1938 FD&C Act defined a "new drug" as any drug which was not generally recognized as safe or as any drug which had become generally recognized as safe but had not been used to a material extent and for a material time. A "generic drug" is a new drug for which approval is sought on the basis of its bioequivalence to a previously approved pioneer new drug and for which no animal or human studies on safety and efficacy were independently conducted [33]. After the DESI project, FDA established their legal position that drugs found to be safe and effective in the DESI review were, in fact, *not* new drugs since they were safe and effective and had been used to a material extent for a material time [34]. Therefore, these drugs were susceptible to classification as generic drugs. Generic manufacturers could gain approval for such generic drugs via an ANDA, as previously described. An ANDA provides a means for a new generic drug to establish that it can provide comparable safety and efficacy to the pioneer drug when the new generic drug is properly manufactured and labeled [34].

Prior to DPC-PTR Act, a generic drug could attain approval either as an ANDA (for drugs approved during the period 1938–1962), a paper NDA (for post-1962 pioneer new drugs), or a full NDA (for post-1962 pioneer new drugs). After the DPC-PTR Act, the ANDA provisions became equally applicable to pioneer drugs approved before 1962 and after 1962. A paper NDA is a full NDA that must satisfy all requirements of a pioneer NDA, but it uses summaries of published studies of animal and human data done by others rather than reports of studies sponsored by the applicant. The key historical events leading to these main provisions of DPC-PTR, as well as other provisions, have been reviewed in detail [35,36] and are summarized in the following sections.

Studies have shown that the effective patent life for pharmaceutical products fell from 13.6 years in 1966 to 9.5 years in 1979 [37-39]. In response to this trend, several bills proposing patent term restoration emerged in the late 1970s. H.R.3589 by Representative Symms (Idaho) was proposed in 1979 to set the patent expiration date for a drug as either 17 years from the date of approval or 27 years from the date of granting patent, whichever was soonest. This legislation failed to gain approval, but did spawn further efforts. In 1980, S.2892 was introduced by Senators Bayh, Thurmond, Mathias, Morgan, and Percy, while H.R.7952 was introduced by Representatives Kastenmeier and Sawyer. These bills contained many of the elements ultimately passed in DPC-PTR. However, no action was taken by that Congress and it was put over to the next session. Modified bills were introduced in the Congress in 1981, but failed to pass due to opposition from groups antagonistic to the research-intensive drug industry.

A report was issued in 1982 after commissioning of research by the Congressional Office of Technology Assessment. This report concluded that patent term restoration could provide incentives to the patent owner to encourage development of new drugs [20]. Senate bill S.255 passed the Senate on July 9, 1981, but the revised counterpart H.R.6444 failed by 5 votes to pass the House on September 15, 1982. This 1982 Patent Term

Restoration Act was defeated, in part, due to the efforts of Representative Henry Waxman (California), then Chairman of the Health Subcommittee of the House Committee on Energy and Commerce. Waxman was interested in providing a mechanism for ANDAs for post-1962 drugs and in assuring that patent term restoration did not severely disadvantage the generic drug companies. Waxman introduced H.R.3605 in 1983 to address the need to apply ANDA regulations to post-1962 drugs. Also in 1983, Senator Mathias led the introduction of S.1306 and Representative Synar (Oklahoma) led the introduction of H.R.3502 as patent term restoration bills. These multiple parties eventually began negotiations wherein the Pharmaceutical Manufacturers Association was represented by PMA president Lewis Engman and general counsel Peter B. Hutt, while the Generic Pharmaceutical Industry Association (GPIA) was represented by GPIA president William Haddad and patent counsel Alfred B. Engelberg. These negotiations ultimately resulted in the DPC-PTR Act as passed in 1984. The extensive negotiations and details of the series of draft bills have been reported elsewhere [35,36,40]. Senator Orrin Hatch (Utah) played an important role as introducer of various Senate bills as Chairman of the hearings by the Senate Committee on Labor and Human Resources. Ultimately, this process led to passage of DPC-PTR.

2. DPC-PTR Provisions for ANDAs and Paper NDAs

It is important to state at the outset that the DPC-PTR Act does not provide restoration of patent term or a market exclusivity period for improvements in a product unless those improvements result in an NDA or supplemental NDA.

The DPC-PTR Act extends the ANDA process to post-1962 drugs. For practical purposes, it is simplest to view the Act as providing for two types of ANDAs, i.e., one type that presents a "generic copy" of a pioneer drug and another type presenting a generic drug that differs from the pioneer drug in some respects. The first type of ANDA follows the same provisions as ANDAs for pre-1962 drugs. Applicants for the second type of ANDA product must first petition FDA for permission to file the ANDA. In granting the petition, FDA may state a requirement for additional information in the ANDA. Alternatively, FDA may reject the petition and direct the applicant to prepare a full NDA.

DPC-PTR also requires applicants for ANDAs to include certification of patent status for any patents listed for the pioneer drug. These certifications are categorized as (1) no patent listed for the pioneer drug, (2) all patents expired for the pioneer drug, (3) all listed patents for the pioneer drug expire on dates provided in the ANDA, (4) patents listed for the pioneer drug are invalid, or (5) patents listed for the pioneer drug will not be infringed by the manufacture and sale of the ANDA drug. If one of the first 3 certifications is stated, the ANDA will be effective upon FDA approval or at the time of patent expiration if that is later than the date of approval. More complicated provisions are in the Act for resolving patent disputes [41].

The DPC-PTR Act defines a paper NDA as one in which the studies used to demonstrate safety and efficacy of the drug "were not conducted by or for the applicant and for which the applicant has not obtained a right of reference or use from the person by or for whom the investigations were conducted " [42]. Peskoe [43] has pointed out that the initial portion of this clause is the same as the original characterization of a paper NDA per Dr. Finkel [31], i.e., that the studies were not conducted by or for the applicant; however, the second clause departs from Dr. Finkel's memorandum by the implication that studies in the public domain can not be used in support of a paper NDA without obtaining a right of reference. Based on this observation, Peskoe [43] argues that since the DPC-PTR Act only recognizes paper NDAs that include a right to reference non-sponsored studies, only such paper NDAs would earn the marketing exclusivity provisions under DPC-PTR. Paper NDAs without right of reference would not be covered under DPC-PTR and, therefore, would earn no exclusivity.

3. DPC-PTR Provisions for Patent Extension

DPC-PTR defines the "regulatory review period" for a human drug as the sum of one-half of the clinical trial period (i.e., the period from IND filing to NDA approval) plus the review period (i.e., the period from NDA filing to NDA approval). DPC-PTR provides for patent extension by the amount of the regulatory review period. The maximum extension is 5 years, but no extension can yield an effective patent life of more than 14 years. However, the Act specifies that the period of patent extension will be decreased by any amount of time during the IND or NDA period that the sponsor did not act with "due diligence." The Act defines due diligence as [44]:

> . . . that degree of attention, continuous directed effort, and timeliness, as may reasonably be expected from, and are ordinarily exercised by, a person during a regulatory review period.

DPC-PTR makes it a responsibility of the sponsor to apply for patent extension within 60 days after approval of the drug. The patents eligible for extension must be identified in the NDA.

DPC-PTR amends one important aspect of patent law. During the life of a patent on a pioneer drug, work done to formulate and test a new generic drug in order to ultimately file an ANDA is not considered an infringement of the pioneer drug patent. Representative Waxman particularly emphasized that this is necessary to assure that when the patent expires for a pioneer drug, competition can begin without delay.

4. DPC-PTR Provisions for Market Exclusivity

The DPC-PTR Act establishes periods of marketing exclusivity for pioneer drugs or significant additions to previously approved drugs in the so-called five exclusivity clauses. Two clauses apply to FDA approvals granted during a pre-enactment period and the other three clauses apply to FDA approvals granted after enactment of DPC-PTR. The exclusivity period is separate from any patent protection and it is operationally imposed by restricting when FDA can approve an ANDA or paper NDA for a generic equivalent of the pioneer drug. These five exclusivity clauses can be summarized as follows [45]:

1. A new chemical entity (NCE) having a full NDA approved between January 1, 1982 and September 24, 1984 received 10 years market exclusivity from the date of NDA approval.
2. A non-NCE product having an NDA or NDA supplement approved for a significant change (e.g., new indication or new route of administration) between January 1, 1982 and September 24, 1984 received market exclusivity until September 24, 1986.
3. All NCEs having an NDA approved after September 24, 1984 receive the following exclusivity:
   a. At least 4 years of market exclusivity is guaranteed. During this period, these NCEs are immune from patent challenge and from generic competition (regardless of patent status).
   b. An unpatented NCE approved after September 24, 1984 will have exclusivity for 5 years plus the time it takes for review and approval at FDA.
   c. An NCE approved after September 24, 1984 with less than 5 years of effective patent life as of the approval date will receive an extension of effective patent life to 5 years.
4. An NDA for a non-NCE that is approved after September 24, 1984 earns market exclusivity only for the nature of the NDA for 3 years from the date of approval only if the NDA contains reports of sponsored new clinical investigations (other than bioavailability studies) essential to approval of the application.
5. An NDA supplement for a non-NCE that is approved after September 24, 1984 earns market exclusivity only for the nature of the supplement (e.g., a new indication) for 3 years from the date

of approval only if the NDA supplement contains reports of sponsored new clinical investigations (other than bioavailability studies) essential to approval of the application.

Interestingly, earning exclusivity for subjects of supplemental NDAs can only be done with "new" clinical trials, i.e., trials not previously submitted to FDA in support of an application.

5. Implications of the DPC-PTR Act

The DPC-PTR Act was one of a series of critical factors contributing to rapid growth in the generic drug industry. Some of the major factors were:

1. Passage of DPC-PTR Act in September 1984
2. Repeal of antisubstitution laws in many states
3. Increased pressure for cost-containment and cost-effective medicines
4. Growing consumer awareness of the availability of generic drugs
5. Growth of the elderly segment of the U.S. population with increasing reliance on drugs for chronic diseases
6. Growth of managed health care systems in the U.S.

Clearly, the generic drug business continues to expand and it has brought more regulatory applications to FDA since the Supreme Court decision that no generic version of a pioneer drug can be marketed without an NDA [46].

The DPC-PTR Act has clear implications for innovation in research-driven pharmaceutical companies. Before DPC-PTR, product development selections were based substantially on the patent protection available for the drug. After DPC-PTR, exclusive product life depends on the applicability of certain provisions to extend the patent term for the drug and provisions to grant certain periods of market exclusivity. It is critical that some drugs may gain market exclusivity under DPC-PTR if the patent has expired or if the product is ineligible for any patent. The latter case can be envisioned to be important to many biotechnology-derived products whose patent status is doubtful.

IX. OTHER MAJOR LEGISLATION

This section provides a brief list of other legislation relevant to certain drug development settings. The Poison Prevention Packaging Act of 1970 requires special packaging to protect children from serious personal injury or illness that could result from handling, using, or ingesting certain household substances, including drugs as defined in the FD&C Act.

Legislation on controlled substances is a separate issue. The original law governing narcotics was the Harrison Narcotic Act of 1914 [47]. This Act attempted to regulate marketing of narcotic drugs by imposing taxes. It did establish a stricter system of control to reduce abuse of the soothing syrups. In 1965, the Drug Abuse Control Amendments were signed into law. These amendments created the BNDD (Bureau of Narcotics and Dangerous Drugs) under the Department of Alcohol, Tobacco, and Firearms. These two major pieces of legislation were joined by approximately 50 other federal laws regulating the handling of narcotics and other substances subject to abuse [11]. In an effort to consolidate effective legislation, the Federal Comprehensive Drug Abuse Prevention and Control Act was enacted in 1970 [48]. Title 2 of this Act is the Controlled Substances Act (CSA). The CSA law is implemented in regulations of the Drug Enforcement Administration (DEA), an agency established within the Department of Justice in July, 1973.

The Drug Listing Act of 1972 requires each manufacturer to maintain with FDA a current listing of each drug it manufactures.

The Orphan Drug Act was signed into law on January 4, 1983 by President Reagan. As other historical legislation, it was co-sponsored by Senator Orrin Hatch and Congressman Henry Waxman. The main elements of this law and a list of orphan drugs have been presented elsewhere [49-51]. This Act fosters a variety of methods and incentives to encourage sponsors to develop and seek approval for orphan drugs, i.e., drugs targeted for a disease affecting less than 200,000 Americans. One estimate is that there are 2,000 such orphan diseases. In fact, in the U.S., there are less than 50,000 patients for most orphan diseases. In 1984, the Act was amended to extend the definition of orphan drugs to include "economic orphans," i.e., diseases in more than 200,000 patients when the sponsor has no reasonable prospect of recovering the research and development costs based on future sales in the U.S.

The Orphan Drug Act describes 18 categories of potential orphan drugs. It offers a means of obtaining a tax credit for a portion of the clinical research needed to support approval. Further, a 7 year period of market exclusivity (regardless of patent status) will be granted to the sponsor after approval by FDA. It is also possible that a more focused preclinical program (e.g., more limited pharmacology and toxicology studies) can be agreed between FDA and sponsor to be adequate. FDA even has a means to contribute limited financial support to defray the cost of the sponsor's clinical research program.

X. SUMMARY

The intent of this chapter was to impress the reader with the relative
youth of legislation governing development and marketing of drugs within
the United States. Less than 100 years ago (in 1906) the first major legislation (Pure Food and Drugs Act) was passed which prohibited interstate
commerce in misbranded or adulterated products, as well as providing
initial recognition of two formal compendia. It was not until 1938 with the
introduction of the FD&C Act that predistribution clearance for safety of
new compounds was required. Separate categorization of legend drugs was
introduced in 1951 with passage of the Durham-Humphrey Amendments.
Prior to that time, a broad spectrum of drugs (e.g., narcotics and antibacterial agents) were available for self-medication without a clear requirement
for adequate directions for use. 1962 brought approval of the Kefauver-
Harris amendments with the initial requirement (only 29 years ago!) for
substantial evidence comprising proof of efficacy prior to distribution of
prescription and non-prescription drugs within the United States. These
amendments led to definition of the nature of clinical investigations as
adequate and well controlled as essential to support approval of applications. Proposed regulations regarding conduct of adequate and well-controlled trials by the sponsor/monitor and investigator were first formalized
in 1977. Within the last five years, we have observed major overhauls of
the regulations regarding investigational and new drug applications. The
necessity for rapid drug development followed by efficient and thorough
review of applications on certain new compounds (e.g., to treat HIV infection) will undoubtedly necessitate further legislative advances affecting
drug review.

It is interesting to note that, prior to passage of the DPC-PTR Act,
all major federal legislation in this area followed a precipitating public
health crisis involving drug-related injury to patients. For example, the
exilir sulfanilamide disaster preceded the 1938 FD&C Act and the thalidomide crisis preceded the 1962 Kefauver-Harris amendments. With
DPC-PTR in 1984 and subsequent federal legislation, there have continued
to be precipitating public health crises. However, these crises have not
involved direct drug-related injury, but rather economic and sociopolitical
crises of inadequate or unequal access to drug therapy. For example, prior
to DPC-PTR, the lack of a systematic pathway for some generic drugs to
gain approval was a major obstacle to the public's option to seek these
drugs. Similarly, passage of the Orphan Drug Act was preceded by a
relative lack of effort by sponsors to develop drugs for patients with orphan
diseases. Finally, recent congressional hearings and pending legislation
focus on a possible law requiring that patients (covered by certain federal

health care programs) have low-cost access to drugs covered by such federal programs. This shift toward economic and sociopolitical motivations, rather than new protections from drug-related injuries, is expected to continue as the predecessor to future federal legislation.

REFERENCES

1. Young JH. The regulation of health quackery. *Pharm. Hist. 26*: 3–12 (1984).
2. Thomas L. *The Youngest Science. Notes of a Medicine-Watcher.* New York: Viking Press, 1983, pp. 19–20.
3. Miller LC. The official compendia—their origins and future. *Amer. J. Pharm. Sci. Supporting Public Health 138*: 175–182 (1966).
4. Janssen WF. Pharmacy and the food and drug law. A significant relationship. *American Pharmacy NS21*: 28–36 (April, 1981).
5. Janssen WF. America's first food and drug laws. *FDA Consumer 9*: 12–18 (June, 1975).
6. Adulteration of drugs. *American Journal of Pharmacy 15*: 382–384 (1849).
7. Wilson S. *Food and Drug Regulations.* Washington, D.C.: American Council on Public Affairs, 1942, pp. 14, 22, 57, 130–131.
8. Janssen WF. The squad that ate poison. *FDA Consumer 15* (No. 10): 6–11 (Dec. 1981–Jan. 1982).
9. History of Drug Regulation. *GMP Reports 1* (No.1), 1979.
10. Sinclair U. *The Jungle.* New York: Signet (reprinted 1960; original publication 1905).
11. Kaluzny E. *Pharmacy Law Digest.* Milwaukee: Douglas-McKay, 1974, pp. 166.14–166.16.
12. Ballentine C. Taste of raspberries, taste of death: the 1937 elixir sulfanilamide incident. *FDA Consumer 15* (No. 5): 18–21 (June, 1981).
13. Hayes AH. Food and drug regulation after 75 years. *JAMA 246*: 1223–1226 (1981).
14. U.S. vs. Sullivan, 332 U.S. 633 (1948).
15. Janssen WF. Outline of the history of U.S. drug regulation and labeling. *Food Drug Cosmetic Law Journal*, pp. 420–441, August, 1981.
16. Florence AL. Is thalidomide to blame? *Brit. Med. J. 2*: 1954 (1960).
17. Fullerton PM, Kremer M. Neuropathy after intake of thalidomide (Distaval). *Brit. Med. J. 2*: 855–858 (1961).
18. Asbury CH. *Orphan Drugs. Medical versus Market Value.* Lexington, KY: D.C. Heath and Co., 1985, page 26.
19. 412 U.S. at 630.
20. Congressional Office of Technology Assessment. *Patent Term Extension and The Pharmaceutical Industry*, 1982.
21. National Academy of Sciences. *Drug Efficacy Study. A Report to the Commissioner of Food and Drugs.* Washington, D.C., 1969.
22. Bryan PA. DESI fifteen years later. *Clin. Res. Practices Drug Reg. Affairs 1*: 241–251 (1983).

23. Mullan PA. Winding down the DESI review. *American Pharmacy NS21* (No. 2): 25–28 (1981).
24. Rogart ME. Paper NDAs and ANDAs for post-1962 drugs—the pioneer manufacturer's view. *Food Drug Cosmetic Law Journal 36*: 129–152 (1981).
25. Vodra WW. Paper NDAs and real problems. *Food Drug Cosmetic Law Journal 39*: 356–384 (1984).
26. Regulations for the enforcement of the Federal Food, Drug, and Cosmetic Act and the Fair Packaging and Labeling Act. *Federal Register 39*: 44602–44657 (1974).
27. Single-entity coronary vasodilators. *Federal Register 42*: 43127–43131 (1977).
28. New policy concerning drugs allowed to remain on market pending completion of studies of effectiveness ("Paragraph XIV" Drugs). *Federal Register 43*: 7044–7045 (1978).
29. Conditions for marketing new drugs evaluated in drug efficacy study. Drugs for human use; Drug Efficacy Study Implementation. *Federal Register 35*: 11273–11274 (1970).
30. Regulations for the enforcement of the Federal Food, Drug, and Cosmetic Act and the Fair Packaging and Labeling Act. *Federal Register 39*: 44634 (1974).
31. Finkel MJ. Memorandum of July 31, 1978: NDA's for Duplicate Drug Products of Post-1962 Drugs. *Federal Register 46*: 27396–27397 (1981).
32. 21 CFR 314.111(a)(5)(ii) (1983).
33. Flannery EJ, Hutt PB. Balancing competition and patent protection in the drug industry: the Drug Price Competition and Patent Term Restoration Act of 1984. *Food Drug Cosmetic Law Journal 40*: 269–309 (1985).
34. Conditions for marketing human prescription drugs. Proposed rule making and notice of enforcement policy for drugs subject to the effectiveness requirements of the Drug Amendments of 1962. *Federal Register 40*: 26142–26156 (1975).
35. Lourie AD. A political history of patent term restoration. Parts I and II. *Pharmaceutical Executive*, pp. 46–48 in January 1985 and pp. 44–54 in February 1985.
36. Lourie AD. Patent term restoration: history, summary, and appraisal. *Food Drug Cosmetic Law Journal 40*: 351–362 (1985).
37. Eisman MM, Wardell WM. The decline in effective patent life of new drugs. *Research Management 21*: 18–21 (1981).
38. Lis Y, Walker SR. Pharmaceutical patent term erosion—A comparison of the UK, the USA and the Federal Republic of Germany. *The Pharmaceutical Journal*, pp. 176–180 (February 6, 1988).
39. Spivey RN, Trimble AG. Effect of the Drug Price Competition Act on market exclusivity of new drugs: a simulation. *Drug Info. J. 20*: 27–35 (1986).
40. Lourie AD. Patent term restoration. *J. Pat. Off. Society 66*,526–66,550 (1984).
41. Shacknai J, Fisher FM. The ANDA/patent extension law: what lies within. *Pharmaceutical Executive*, pp. 36–44, January 1985.
42. Public Law No. 98–417, article 103(a).

43. Peskoe MP. Paper NDAs and the Drug Price Competition Act: a last hurrah? *Food Drug Cosmetic Law Journal 40*: 323–328 (1985).
44. Kaplan A, Becker R. ANDA/patent extension balancing act. *Pharmaceutical Executive*, pp. 58–62, February 1985.
45. Pape SM. Market exclusivity under the Drug Price Competition and Patent Term Restoration Act of 1984—the five clauses. *Food Drug Cosmetic Law Journal 40*: 310–316 (1985).
46. U.S. versus Generix Drug Corp., 460 U.S. 453, 1983.
47. Former 21 U.S.C. 4701 et seq.
48. 21 U.S.C. 801 et seq.
49. Spilker B. Development of orphan drugs. *Trends in Pharmacological Sciences 6*: 185–188 (1985).
50. Weck E. Medicine's 'orphans': drugs for rare diseases. *FDA Consumer 22* (No. 1): 12–14 (February, 1988).
51. Food and Drug Administration. Cumulative list of orphan-drug and biological designations. *Federal Register 54*: 7100–7108 (February 16, 1989).

12

The Present: Current Trends and Controversies

> I find the great thing in this world is
> not so much where we stand as in what
> direction we are moving.
>
> *Oliver Wendell Holmes*

I. INTRODUCTION

This chapter was formulated intentionally as a collection of observations and comments on miscellaneous topics that were current during the time of its writing. We do not portend to foresee all of the patterns in these events; we leave expanded interpretation to the reader.

II. INDUSTRIAL CONSOLIDATION

Any chapter on current trends and controversies in drug development must begin with recognition of industrial consolidation. Consolidation within the pharmaceutical industry began to occur more commonly in the early 1980s and it became a very active trend in the late 1980s. The year 1989 saw mergers of Squibb with Bristol-Myers, Smith Kline with Beecham, and Marion Laboratories with Merrell Dow. These and other examples of consolidations are listed in Table 1. Certainly, the large investment needed to sustain productivity in diverse R&D areas is one reason for such mergers [1,2]. One pharmaceutical industry executive estimated that it takes in excess of $200 million in R&D expenditure/year to compete in the arena of new chemical entity development [1]. One author speculated that the

194

Table 1. Corporate parties to various pharmaceutical industry mergers, consolidations, buyouts, and joint ventures.

First Party	Second Party	Resultant Company (if a new name applies)
American Critical Care	DuPont	DuPont Critical Care
American Home Products	A.H. Robins	
Key Laboratories	Schering-Plough	Schering-Plough
Marion	Merrell Dow	Marion Merrell Dow
Merck	DuPont	DuPont-Merck
Meyer Laboratories	Glaxo Group Limited	Glaxo Inc.
Parke Davis	Warner Lambert	
Pennwalt	Fisons	Fisons
Roche Holdings	Genentech, Inc.	
Rorer Group	Rhone-Poulenc S.A.	
G.D. Searle	Monsanto	
Smith Kline	Beecham	SmithKline Beecham
Squibb Corp.	Bristol-Myers Co.	Bristol-Myers Squibb
Sterling Drug	Eastman Kodak	Eastman Kodak Co.
Wyeth	Ayerst	Wyeth-Ayerst Laboratories

dramatic increases in the cost of innovation is the strongest single factor fueling consolidation [2].

Another type of consolidation is the potential for business and regulatory consolidation as a result of approaching changes in the European Community in 1992. Although the possibilities presented by this change remain to be fully elucidated, European consolidation has the potential to dramatically alter the regulatory aspects of clinical drug development in affected European countries.

III. INTERNATIONAL USES OF CLINICAL TRIAL DATA

Clinical trial data generated outside the United States are increasingly submitted as a component of evidence of safety and efficacy in a new drug application filed in the U.S. This is a more subtle example of industrial consolidation. The role of data collected in foreign clinical trials (not conducted under an IND) has evolved separately for safety data versus efficacy data. Since the IND rewrites became effective, safety data has become universal, i.e., all safety data from all clinical trials, regardless of the country of origin, are susceptible to reporting within the United States under the relevant IND. The frequency and detail of safety reports increase as the degree of seriousness increases. This is another example of the sliding scale concept discussed in Chapter 5. The extreme example of safety reporting is foreign data reportable as IND Safety Reports since these data must be the subject of either a 3-day or 10-day report to FDA with appropriate informative correspondence sent to all investigators active under the IND. Other foreign safety data must be reported either in periodic progress reports to the IND or a safety update, as appropriate.

Efficacy data collected in foreign clinical trials is not used in as certain a manner as safety data. The greater flexibility for efficacy data is an accommodation to the different arts of the practice of medicine from country to country. For example, a company developing an antibiotic for both oral and parenteral administration may choose to use foreign clinical trials to focus solely on the parenteral form in certain countries (e.g., Italy) where parenteral drugs are more commonly prescribed for out-patients. A second example is the relatively sparse use of spirometric measures of pulmonary function in studies of a new bronchodilator in most European trials, compared with serial intra-day measures via spirometry as a primary quantitative index of efficacy for studies done within the U.S. As long as these differences in medical research practices persist, the achievable extent of internationalization of clinical efficacy studies will continue to be drug specific. Several drugs have been approved in the U.S. based on New Drug Applications containing pivotal data from foreign studies (Table 2).

These examples of uses of safety and efficacy data to support multinational regulatory applications have led some authors to summarize

Table 2. Drugs approved in the U.S. using primary evidence from foreign clinical studies.

Drugs Approved Based *Solely* on Non-U.S. Pivotal Studies:	
Blockadren	(timolol; sNDA for prevention of reinfarction; MSD)
Cyklokapron	(tranexamic acid; KabiVitrum)
Haldol Decanoate	(haloperidol; McNeil)
Mesnex	(mesna; Bristol-Myers)
Drugs Approved Based on Pivotal U.S. and Non-U.S. Studies:	
Buspar	(buspirone; Mead Johnson)
Losec	(omeprazole; MSD)
Marinol	(dronabinol; Roxane)
Nimotop	(nimodipine; Miles)
Nolvadex	(tamoxifen; ICI)
Zofran	(ondansetron; Glaxo)

Source: Ref. 3.

FDA's particular concerns about data collected outside the United States. Some of these concerns are (1) the potential medical, genetic, and cultural differences between the study population and the U.S. patient population; (2) the FDA's relative unfamiliarity with the training, experience, and facilities of foreign clinical investigators; (3) FDA's restricted ability to conduct on-site inspections of foreign clinical investigators; and (4) lack of certification of some foreign clinical laboratories [4-6]. Clearly, companies moving toward extensive internationalization of clinical drug development must prospectively build responses to these concerns into their drug development plans.

IV. CONTRACT RESEARCH ORGANIZATIONS

The role of contract research organizations (CRO) has evolved rapidly. With respect to clinical drug development, federal regulations define a CRO as ". . . a person that assumes, as an independent contractor with the sponsor, one or more of the obligations of a sponsor, e.g., design of a protocol, selection or monitoring of investigations, evaluation of reports, and preparation of materials to be submitted to the Food and Drug Administration" [7]. The IND rewrite introduced the requirement that a sponsor specifically identify those regulatory obligations of the sponsor that are transferred to the CRO. This requirement seemingly would make sponsors consider carefully which obligations on which projects should be completed by a CRO; some people speculated that the extent of contracting might diminish over time. Although increased care of consideration appears to have happened in many sponsoring organizations, the latter business constriction has not happened. The total number of CROs has increased in the last ten years. Further, there are several CROs that now have experience executing clinical drug development plans and preparing a NDA for a new chemical entity. These trends appear to be continuing as more sponsors use more CRO services in an effort to increase productivity of clinical research without increasing intracompany resources and without incurring the training-associated delays that occur when hiring new, inexperienced personnel.

Of particular significance to us is the trend over the past few years for CROs to hire senior personnel with industry-wide and nationwide scientific repute. Certainly, 15 years ago, few of us knew many CRO-employed clinical scientists who were widely known and respected. Today, there are many well recognized clinical scientists on the staffs of CROs. This change seems consistent with the increasing acceptance of the role of CROs in clinical drug development. Indeed, this acceptance has become reliance for some sponsors.

V. R&D PRODUCTIVITY

The desire to measure R&D productivity at many companies is consistent with the desire to apply conventional project management approaches to clinical drug development. Both productivity measurement and conventional forms of project management assume that the process being measured and managed is resource limited. Information in several earlier chapters argues that the innovative clinical drug development process is intellect limited. Nonetheless, various industry watchers (e.g., drug stock analysts) continue in their efforts to measure R&D productivity. One of the most recent efforts was reported in January 1989 [1]. That study used indices such as new sales/R&D spending, R&D spending/total sales, and new sales/equity for 12 companies that are very active in the U.S. Such indices do not allow for capture of cost of R&D traceable to a specific line of research due to the time displacement of drug approval and sale from the time of R&D expenditure. Further, these indices do not include some reflection of the likelihood of success of the investigational drugs still in the pipelines, nor do they measure the likely therapeutic importance of the drug, value of research equity generated by various projects, or the likely FDA response to pending NDAs.

The drive to measure R&D productivity is one factor moving companies to more targeted drug development programs. Such programs may be more predictable with respect to productivity. It may also be a factor that drives companies to smooth their financial performance charts through consolidation efforts. Our concern is the lack of evidence that efforts to measure R&D productivity are related in some manner to enhanced R&D productivity. It is difficult to envision a productivity index that could incorporate measures of the spontaneous discovery and quantum leaps of knowledge that are characteristic of true research intellects [8].

VI. OPERATING TRENDS AT FDA

FDA has tried consistently and continues to try to become more interactive without sacrificing efficient use of time. This trend is reflected in the recent Subpart E regulations wherein a means is provided for FDA to meet with the sponsor early, relatively often, and with a detailed agenda in order to design and execute a mutually agreeable drug development plan. Such a plan gives the drug the potential to attain approval after a minimum of adequate and well-controlled studies [9]. Other examples are provided by the various drugs approved for treatment use under a treatment IND or treatment protocol following active interchange between FDA and sponsor. Opportunities for these types of exchanges must continue to be available with time allocated in a prioritized manner to drugs with the greatest potential therapeutic impact.

A trend related to the interactive style of FDA is the introduction of so-called "NDA days." On this day, the reviewing division at FDA reviews and questions in detail the observations in an NDA, while representatives of the sponsor may be present to provide immediate responses to concerns. Such efforts can provide a means to rapidly dispose of lesser issues amenable to simple explanation and focus the review on any major issues that remain for discussion. Some divisions at FDA have used this approach successfully [10-12]. This type of approach is consistent with availability of newer tools (e.g., computer-assisted NDAs and optical disk NDAs) that facilitate rapid access to information and some query capabilities.

VII. GENERIC DRUGS

The volatile generic drug controversy [13,14] that resulted in criminal convictions in 1989 and 1990 was the result, ultimately, of an increasingly deregulated environment. A careful reading of the previous chapter on the history of laws governing drug development in the U.S. reveals that this outcome for generic drugs is not surprising. There are numerous historical parallels where health quackery emerged in a setting of inadequate regulatory controls.

Clearly, there is a major role for generic drugs in assuring competitive pricing and cost-effective drug products for American patients. This assurance, however, must be provided through development, manufacture, sale, and distribution of generic drugs of demonstrated quality and therapeutic equivalence to the standard pioneer product. These latter standards can only be maintained by companies committed to quality and efficient regulatory monitoring via a FDA equipped with adequate resources to execute these tasks efficiently.

VIII. SHIFTING NATURE OF PATIENT POPULATIONS

Several patient-related trends have been developing for many years. One trend is the increasing definition of more narrowly defined patient subpopulations and narrowly specified indications for new drugs. For example, the reader can compare the rather broad wording of the indications for the older antibiotic Amoxil® with the newer antibiotic Augmentin® from the same company. The more specific wording is due in part to the need to specify a subpopulation of patients for this drug and to carefully define each indication. The H-2 antagonists (Tagamet®, Zantac®, Pepcid®, Axid®) provide interesting examples of some drugs approved for short-term treatment versus maintenance therapy for gastric ulcer or duodenal ulcer or GERD. Each specific indication carries restrictions on the target patient subpopulation in recognition that each such subpopulation may have a different benefit/risk profile with each drug. These trends toward more specific labeling are visible evidence of the preference to individualize treatment of the individual patient.

The second trend is the shift in demographic characteristics of the population of the United States toward the elderly. This trend has implications for the types and frequencies of diseases encountered, dose-response characteristics, safety of drugs, and a host of other factors. Such major demographic trends require attention in drug development programs. It is judicious to anticipate future regulations that necessitate special attention to this age group in clinical drug development programs.

The third trend is that drugs are being developed predominantly for episodic and chronic diseases. These latter diseases introduce the need to evaluate the efficacy of intermittent and continuous maintenance therapies, as well as the increasing need for long-term safety data in man.

IX. DEMONSTRATING IMPROVED QUALITY OF LIFE AS A PRECURSOR TO DRUG APPROVAL

There is a clear trend toward more widespread use of measures of quality of life as a component of the clinical drug development and approval process. This trend to measure the patient's perception of the extent to which the patient feels better and maintains an unimpaired lifestyle has accompanied the shift in focus from acute diseases to episodic and chronic diseases. For example, the long-term impact of an acute urinary tract infection on a patient's quality of life does not seem as inherently critical compared with the impact of lifelong therapy for hypertension. Research on characterizing the degree of disease-associated impairment in quality-of-life measures is perhaps best illustrated by the Medical Outcomes Study [15,16].

An excellent overview of the general principles of quality of life assessment was provided by Miller et al. [17]. A more detailed text is available [18]. Miller et al. [19] have also provided guidance specifically with respect to oncology drugs. For these and several other classes of drugs, quality of life indices have proven useful as one index of the treatment-associated reduction in morbidity. This is particularly helpful in detecting differential activity of the drug when other, more conventional measures of efficacy may be only marginally sensitive to intertreatment differences in long-term effects of the drug. For example, the often-cited study of captopril versus methyldopa versus propranolol showed all three drugs to be effective in reducing diastolic blood pressure. The mean 24-week diastolic blood pressures were 87.1, 87.7, and 86.1 mm Hg in the captopril, methyldopa, and propranolol groups, respectively [20]. In contrast to these relatively small and statistically insignificant differences in this conventional index of efficacy, captopril was associated with significantly greater improvements in several measures of quality of life [20]. This study shows the type of important information that can be collected by using selected validated quality of life instruments in clinical trials. Although the role of such data as a determinant of drug approval is not yet clear for many drug classes, it is clear that several reviewing divisions at FDA recognize the potentially important information provided by these instruments and they have encouraged their use as a contributing component to the panel of measures of a new drug's safety and efficacy.

REFERENCES

1. Teitelman R, Baldo A. Grading R&D. *Financial World*, pp. 22–24 (January 24, 1989).
2. *The Pharmaceutical Industry: Trade Related Issues*. Paris: Organisation for Economic Co-operation and Development, 1985, p. 26.
3. Lisook AB. FDA audits of clinical studies: policy and procedure. *J. Clin. Pharmacol. 30*: 296–302 (1990).
4. Hurley FL. Planning research and development of new drugs to assure regulatory approval. *Food Drug Cosmetic Law Journal 39*: 312–317 (1984).
5. Fredd SB. FDA's regulation of foreign clinical data on new drugs. 26th Annual Meeting of the Drug Information Association. San Francisco, CA. June 5, 1990.
6. Honohan T. Practical problems in the conduct of non-US studies from which data will be used for US registration. *Drug Information Journal 22*: 193–197 (1988).
7. New drug, antibiotic, and biologic drug product regulations; final rule. Section 312.3. Definitions and interpretations. *Federal Register 52* (Number 53): 8798–8847 (1987).
8. Kuhn TS. *The Structure of Scientific Revolutions*. Chicago: University of Chicago Press, p. 75, 1970.
9. Investigational New Drug, Antibiotic, and Biological Drug Product Regulations; Subpart E—Procedures for Drugs Intended to Treat Life-Threatening and Severely Debilitating Illnesses. *Federal Register 53* (No. 204): 41516–41524 (October 21, 1988).
10. Upjohn Ansaid "NDA-Day" accelerated review 3–6 months, firm estimates; FDA's Temple says scheduling function is key to time savings with NDA-Days. *F-D-C Reports (The Pink Sheet) 51*: 6–7 (June 26, 1989).
11. FDA's first open "NDA-day". *Scrip World Pharmaceutical News*, No. 1444, p. 18 (September 6, 1989).

12. "NDA Day" planned for novel dosage form of previously approved ingredient. *F-D-C Reports (The Pink Sheet)* 52: T&G-4 (May 21, 1990).
13. Freudenheim M. A confident generics industry. Long-term growth seen despite inquiry. *The New York Times*, August 18, 1989.
14. Ingersoll B. FDA finds problems at 10 of 12 firms being probed in generic-drug scandal. *The Wall Street Journal*, September 12, 1989.
15. Stewart AL, Greenfield S, Hays RD, Wells K, Rogers WH, Berry SD, McGlynn EA, Ware JE. Functional status and well-being of patients with chronic conditions. Results from the Medical Outcomes Study. *JAMA 262*: 907–913 (1989).
16. Wells KB, Stewart A, Hays RD, Burnam MA, Rogers W, Daniels M, Berry S, Greenfield S, Ware J. The functioning and well-being of depressed patients. Results from the Medical Outcomes Study. *JAMA 262*: 914–919 (1989).
17. Miller L, Dalton M, Vestal R, Perkins JG, Lyon G. Quality of Life. I. Methodological and regulatory/scientific aspects. *J. Clin. Res. Drug Development 3*: 117–128 (1989).
18. Spilker B, ed. *Quality of Life Assessments in Clinical Trials*. New York: Raven Press, 1990.
19. Miller L, Vestal R, Dalton M, Atwood B, Perkins JG, Lyon G. Quality of Life. II. Oncology: regulatory/scientific aspects and the drug approval process. *J. Clin. Res. Pharmacoepidemiology 4*: 39–53 (1990).
20. Croog SH, Levine S, Testa MA, Brown B, Bulpitt CJ, Jenkins CD, Klerman GL, Williams GH. The effects of antihypertensive therapy on the quality of life. *N. Engl. J. Med. 314*: 1657–1664 (1986).

13

The Future of Clinical Drug Development

He who does not go forward goes backward.

Johann Wolfgang von Goethe

I. INTRODUCTION

The opening quotation is applicable to the pharmaceutical industry; a company must go forward to avoid going backward since it is simply not possible to stay in a fixed location relative to an ever-changing business, research, and medical environment. This book has focused on the key scientific and management issues that must be addressed to go forward in the clinical drug development process. We have discussed how management can use critical mass research teams to foster the type of teamwork and research capabilities necessary to perform studies yielding *decision-enabling* data. These sections have argued that clinical drug development should not merely be an exercise in "regulatory hurdle jumping." Indeed, if discovery and development of new drugs are pursued as a research exercise focused on sound scientific evaluation of new chemical entities, then the regulatory hurdles will be jumped and the knowledge generated in the process will actually contribute to corporate research equity.

The last three chapters of this book were collected as a unit in order to provide a detailed perspective on the historical legal and regulatory environment for clinical drug development in the United States, followed by a commentary on some current issues and controversies, and, finally, the future of drug discovery and development. There are two global aspects of the future. The first global aspect is the *regulatory and corporate environment* of drug development. The second global aspect is the *opportunities* that will present themselves in the future. In this chapter, we will attempt to outline some of the details of these global aspects of the future. We will not attempt to enumerate a list of specific drug development opportunities for reasons that will become apparent.

Consider first the environment in which drug development will be conducted in the future. We consider environment first because the environment will actually influence the opportunities that drug developers will pursue.

II. REGULATORY ENVIRONMENT

Consider the regulatory environment from the point of view of the regulator. Basically, the FD&C Act, its amendments, and their implementation described in the *Code of Federal Regulations* require that the regulator attempt to assess whether the benefit/risk ratio for any new chemical entity is greater than one, that is, the benefits outweigh the risks, for the specific proposed use of the drug. We can illustrate this decision-making process as an assessment of where the drug fits on a number line measuring various benefit/risk ratios (Figure 1). Ratios greater than 1 indicate a drug in the approvable range and ratios less than 1 are clearly in the non-approvable range. Ratios exactly equal to one would fall in the non-approvable range, except in rare instances (e.g., an otherwise untreatable disease) where trading equal benefits for equal risks might be approvable.

A. Discerning Drugs that are Potentially Approvable

The regulatory review process would be easy if it were possible to place an "X" on the number line to accurately represent the benefit/risk ratio for a new drug. Unfortunately, the benefit/risk assessment is usually not

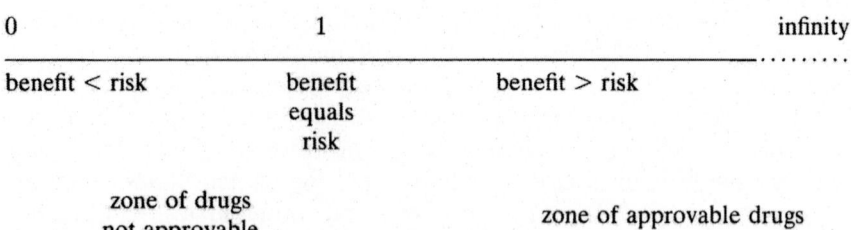

Figure 1. Number line of benefit/risk ratios.

a simple quantitative ratio for all patients, especially in view of the heterogeneity among patients who are candidates for this new therapy. Thus, the benefit/risk assessment actually yields a range. This *range of benefit/risk ratio* is the natural result of the sliding scale which we have discussed previously; it is the *range of minimum to maximum achievable benefit per unit risk.* The biological basis for this range is variability among patients. In brief, not all patients with a given disease have equivalent disease-associated morbidity and mortality. Consequently, the possible benefit of treatment is not uniform across all patients. Similarly, not all patients experience the same drug-associated risk from a given therapy; consequently, the drug-associated risk is not uniform across all patients.

Two regulatory/scientific judgements must be made in order to determine whether or not a new chemical entity is approvable: (1) how broad is this range of benefit/risk ratios and (2) where is the range located on the number line? The regulations require that regulators approve drugs for use in specific indications only where the benefits outweigh the risks. Thus, if the benefit/risk ratio is clearly greater than 1 for all patient populations studied, the decision to approve the drug appears quite straightforward. Similarly, if the benefit/risk ratio is clearly less than 1 for some or many populations treated with the new chemical entity, then the drug should not and will not be approved for this use. Obviously, the closer the range of benefit/risk ratios is to 1, the more difficult the decision-making process becomes. In such cases, the regulator must assess whether or not a portion or most of this range actually extends below 1. From the regulatory viewpoint, it is not prudent to approve drugs with a significant chance of having a benefit/risk ratio below one in the target patient population. Thus, the drug approval process can be facilitated by demonstrating either that the benefit/risk ratio range is much greater than 1 or by demonstrating that the benefit/risk ratio range is fairly narrow and only slightly greater than 1.

It is not uncommon for an original NDA to consist of a mixture of different populations of patients that yielded a broad range of benefit/risk ratios around the value 1. Such a drug may be approvable if separate re-analyses of the individual subpopulations reveal one or more approvable subpopulations with ranges of benefit/risk ratios greater than 1 versus one or more different, non-approvable subpopulations with benefit/risk ratios less than 1. The approvable subpopulations can be carefully described in restrictive labeling for the approvable product.

B. Applicability of the NDA Data to the Post-Approval Patient Population

The preceding considerations can lead the regulator to the conclusion that a new drug is potentially approvable based on the evidence of a favorable benefit/risk ratio in the clinical trial population. However, the regulator must then escalate evaluation of the drug to the next level by assessing whether the findings in the pre-approval clinical drug trials can be generalized to the usually broader, more heterogeneous population that will use the drug after approval. One reason for the NDA rewrites was the concern that data submitted in NDAs typically report only narrow subpopulations within a given disease population. Such data may not be predictive of the broader population. The NDA rewrites encourage increased post-marketing surveillance of new chemical entities as they enter broader patient populations after marketing. This period of post-marketing surveillance would enable the regulatory authorities to assess whether the labeling that was originally approved for a new chemical entity remains appropriate as the drug is used in a more heterogeneous patient population. This concern has been heightened in the competitive marketplace in part by the fact that many companies try to interpret their approved indications for the broadest possible patient population. This is quite understandable from a commercial perspective since it facilitates the broadest use of the drug.

Regulators must continue to wrestle with this issue of appropriate identification of the target patient population even for drugs with large benefit/risk ratios. As the chance of a benefit/risk ratio less than or equal to 1 increases owing to the breadth or position of the benefit/risk range, the approval decision may be delayed in an attempt to allow either additional studies or post-marketing experience in other countries to help define further the benefits and risks of the new chemical entity under review in the U.S. There is every reason to believe that this regulatory perspective will continue in the future. In addition, it is reasonable to expect future regulations and guidelines to require (prior to approval of a new chemical entity) a more precise definition of the target patient population in the proposed labeling for the drug. Ideally, these target populations can be described in the package insert of the new drug based on substantial evidence that these specific populations have favorable benefit/risk ratios.

C. More Specific versus More General Regulations and Guidelines

The FDA is in a position where they must make decisions based on available data. *Regulations cannot dictate the intent of the sponsor, scientific integrity of the clinical research, and accuracy of the benefit/risk assessment*; indirectly, regulations affect these factors by requiring specific types of data. This is indeed a dilemma because the spirit of the FD&C Act and regulations is to address the scientific principles of sound drug development without specifying in detail the data required. This lack of detail is intentional in recognition of the fact that science and the scientific understanding of disease are constantly evolving. We have discussed the dynamic nature of science in previous chapters and we pointed out the potential discontinuities that can befall the sponsor who is not modifying a drug's development plan as new knowledge arises. Some, who view drug development as a series of regulatory hurdles, prefer issuance of more specific regulations and guidelines to prospectively define the location and height of every hurdle. While such a specific "letter of the law" approach might appear to better define the endpoints and facilitate drug development, more specific regulations and guidelines will, in practice, be far more restrictive. Consider that the rate at which scientific understanding about disease and disease mechanisms is increasing easily outstrips our rate of discovering and developing new drugs. This rapid evolution of our medical and scientific databases is one reason that most FDA guidelines for clinical development of specific drug classes are 5 to 15 years old and operationally outdated. Some persons at FDA have recognized that a new guideline will be outdated by the time it can be issued. Consequently, if guidelines were very specific regarding the data required for approval of a new chemical entity, it is unlikely that any future therapies could be fully developed without experiencing at least one change in the regulatory environment. Such changes would be dictated by increased knowledge that would make prior measures of safety and efficacy outdated at best and inappropriate at worst.

Some sponsors and investigators have argued that specific regulations for each drug class would define the endpoint of clinical drug development and assure application of the same standard for all drugs. For example, specific regulations would tell us that an adequate and well-controlled trial of a new anti-hypertensive drug must consist of a randomized (1:1), double-blind, placebo-controlled evaluation of 4-months duration in 140 patients with serial determinations via ambulatory blood pressure monitoring. This view is misguided since a truly equal standard for different drugs already exists in the requirement to form an adequate benefit/risk assessment; mere execution of an identical study design for two drugs may not yield an adequate benefit/risk assessment for each.

D. Future Regulatory Environment

Unfortunately, the interest of simplicity often drives sponsors to explain the regulatory process as a series of hurdles rather than explain the real spirit of the law. History provides examples of some sponsors who violated the letter and spirit of the law. Whenever such violations occur and result in substantial compromise of the public welfare, it leads to new laws, regulations, or guidelines. We see a new round of regulatory action on the horizon; this regulatory action will persist as long as regulatory approval is the primary goal of clinical drug development, rather than a by-product of scientific evaluation of new chemical entities in the interest of aiding the public health. The approaching unification of the European market will continue its recent trend to resemble the FDA from a regulatory perspective. In the next century, it is likely that worldwide regulatory authorities will increase the scope and intensity of reviews, especially for compounds adding little or nothing to the current therapeutic armamentarium.

Thus, we conclude that increasing specificity of regulations and guidelines will actually complicate the drug development process. There are always some individuals who will attempt to subvert the process for financial gain. Such breaches will obviously lead to yet another round of restrictive regulations and intensive inspections by FDA. Thus, it seems quite rational to expect that the regulatory environment will become more inhospitable to drug development, particularly for drugs providing little or no addition to the therapeutic armamentarium. The community of innovative drug developers has a vested interest in attempting to avoid the regulatory-hurdle-jumping mentality. Moreover, the industry must be willing to police itself in order to counter individuals who ultimately effect undesirable changes, while the majority of drug developers are conducting their operations with integrity.

III. CORPORATE ENVIRONMENT

A. Corporate Strategies from Viewing Drug Development as a Series of Regulatory Hurdles

In the corporate drug development environment, the need for coordination between R&D (research and development) and M&S (marketing and sales) has fueled the "project management mentality." This timeline-oriented, resource management system relies on tangible project goals (e.g., filing an NDA). Often, work becomes focused solely on what needs to be done to submit an NDA. Occasionally, the focus goes beyond NDA submission to encompass NDA approval, but rarely would the goal of project management be to understand use of the drug in the target patient population. Obviously, the latter goal is far more difficult to predict and schedule compared with predicting the time to cross a series of predefined regulatory hurdles. Therefore, the tendency has been to define a "letter of the law" resource management approach to the drug development process in order to facilitate "paper" coordination between R&D and M&S. That is, communication and coordination between R&D and M&S *seem* aided by R&D's portrayal of clinical drug development as a resource-limited process amenable to display on a Gantt chart. This approach to drug development can elicit some undesirable responses from regulators as they attempt to ascertain whether clearing all hurdles comprises an adequate scientific evaluation in light of the current understanding of disease. With such an approach, the fundamental responsibility to assure a reasonable and prudent scientific evaluation of new drugs can tacitly become the regulator's responsibility, rather than the responsibility of the sponsor as stated in the regulations.

There are other flaws to the hurdle-jumping approach. As science evolves, the laws and regulations will also change. Therefore, the regulatory environment that was assumed in the initial project management plan will no longer exist by the time a new chemical entity moves from the initial studies in man to a registration document. An even greater longer-term danger exists as preclinical drug discovery research is also being swept into the project management mentality. The current mentality focuses on resource management and the notion that discovering new drugs requires large resources. This large need for resources is one rationale often cited for ongoing consolidation in the industry. Companies are either merging or limiting their work to a few therapeutic areas in order to focus greater resources on more rapid discovery and development of new chemical entities in a more limited arena. Such a focused approach is especially common when the bulk of the research is directed toward producing me-too compounds. As we reported in Chapter 1, the decade of the 1980s saw that almost 60% of the new chemical entities approved were category 1-C compounds. Commonly, such compounds encounter increased regulatory difficulties because the perceived need for such drugs is low. The cost of clinical development of such drugs is increased because of the high cost of finding something to distinguish the compound from the competition, as well as the high cost of generating interest and attention for the compound. Clinical research costs are lower for some drugs with significant therapeutic gain because such prototype compounds often get some independent, "free" research from the scientific community. Me-too compounds may actually receive a "double whammy" because clinical development of the compound would not enable one to provide novel and interesting information about the drug and the disease process, in addition to costing more to find only subtle distinguishing features of the drug. Of course, me-too drug discovery and development is admittedly more predictable when resources are adequate. However, the costs are high and returns are not as large, especially for compounds that are the third or later entry to a given therapeutic area. Despite these disadvantages, the increasingly market-driven nature of the future corporate environment will render it more oriented towards predictable, lower risk research and development. This orientation will result in more segments of the market with multiple "patented generics", much the same as we now have with a large array of marketed beta-blockers and diuretics. It is difficult if not impossible to reap extraordinary returns on such me-too products.

B. Innovative Drug Discovery in Corporations

In the future, truly innovative drug discovery and development will take place outside the traditional pharmaceutical industry. The approximately 11,000 to 12,000 biotechnology-oriented companies that have been started in the last 15 years are evidence that there is money available for promising high-risk ventures in drug discovery and development. Many of these small biotechnology companies can ultimately only distribute their products via the marketing and sales divisions of major pharmaceutical companies. Although this approach will enable such venture-originator products to achieve their full market potential, it will also promote further erosion of the research orientation of the traditional pharmaceutical industry.

Alternatively, the traditional pharmaceutical industry could hold to its research-intensive history by turning away from a predominantly market-driven R&D program to a more scientifically-driven drug discovery and development effort. If this occurs, the corporate R&D environment will become more oriented towards identification of new therapeutic targets. Then, the corporate environment will become one of exploitation of both biotechnology and the traditional pharmaceutical approaches to the discovery and development of new drugs. Such incorporation of new technologies, expansion of research mentality, and avoidance of the "not-invented-here" syndrome is the preferred path to the future.

IV. OPPORTUNITIES

A. The Contrarian Strategy

Future opportunities must be projected in view of the perspective of the future regulatory and corporate environments. Basically, the opportunities lie in a contrarian strategy, i.e., avoiding the present trends of the masses and avoiding the direction suggested by linear extrapolation to the future. The major opportunity lies in not following everyone else. That is, as much as possible try to avoid doing what others are doing because in fact *the objective of R&D is not to create new products that compete with other products, but rather to create products that are unique and innovative and therefore have no competition.* Such innovative products are rewarding in the scientific, medical, and commercial senses. Products with outstanding therapeutic activity and favorable benefit/risk ratios are very rarely commercial disasters. Even a product like misoprostil managed to find a very profitable niche as a preventive agent for NSAID-induced ulceration, despite failure to gain approval for the disease it was initially targeted to treat (i.e., duodenal ulcer disease).

Clearly, the path less traveled is not without risk. However, the potential for higher reward generally requires higher risk and, conversely, the path of low risk and predictable outcomes usually yields only modest returns (at best!). The future lies in identification of unique opportunities. Drug discovery and development is a research endeavor with a unifying research process and mentality. Attention must be focused on quality and innovation in both discovery and development of new drugs.

B. Maximum Value from the Research Information Base

We must develop a means to value and exploit research information as highly as we ultimately exploit the products of research. Failure to exploit our own research-information base has been one reason for U.S. lag in international competitiveness. Some of our foreign competitors aggressively exploit the U.S. research-information base. This information base is the key to identification of new opportunities. Products will arise from this information as a by-product of careful, thoughtful, and aggressive consideration of this information in concert with discovery and development research. The success of the Japanese in applying American information to development of new products in several industries is a shining example of this principle in action.

C. Identification of New Therapeutic Targets

Occasionally, we hear that many of the "easy" products have already been developed and consequently future drug development will be far more difficult. In fact, the biotechnology revolution argues strongly against this assessment. Development of new ligands is virtually limitless in the context of biotechnology, organic synthesis, and the combination of the two. Rather, the difficulty lies in identification of targets for these products. As many biotechnology companies have learned, it is necessary but not sufficient to be able to generate pharmacologically active moieties. If understanding of the disease and consequently selection of the target does not improve, then the biotechnology industry will produce a series of TPA-like episodes in which a compound achieves objective commercial success, but ultimately fails to achieve success in the eyes of the corporation because its sales are only a fraction of the company's original expectation. We must focus more on identification of therapeutic targets as one of the products of R&D. Similarly, evaluation of therapeutic targets must also be one of the systematic endeavors of R&D. Maximum value from the research information base can be achieved in part by using information in one field of research to identify potential new targets in a different field of research. If we are able to identify new research targets and therapeutic opportunities, then the tools of biotechnology and traditional organic synthesis become the means to exploit our new-found understanding for scientific, medical, and commercial success.

This line of thought may lead some major pharmaceutical companies toward a strict therapeutic orientation. For example, a company could evolve such that they focus on understanding viral diseases and develop products for treatment of viral diseases. This company would not only develop new therapies, but would also exploit the information obtained in their research endeavors to develop diagnostic products and possibly even new technological approaches for research in that therapeutic area. Such a company would probably establish loose ties with research-oriented, technology-based companies and marketing relationships with partners with the capabilities to optimize the marketing effort and optimize return for any new discoveries. Collaborative relationships might also be established with academic centers with high expertise in this specific research area.

One shortcoming of a company with a therapeutic orientation is that it will be increasingly difficult to find application for their research discoveries with potential uses outside the chosen therapeutic area. This creates one final longer term opportunity for those select few large pharmaceutical firms that remain oriented towards research-driven drug development. Such firms can develop very broad research capabilities and collaborative agreements that enable them to work effectively across multiple therapeutic categories. Their products will then be sold either directly or with the aid of co-marketing agreements. This small cadre of integrated research-oriented pharmaceutical companies will distance themselves from both the smaller research-oriented companies that emerge and the market-oriented companies which remain from the present pharmaceutical industry. These large integrated research-oriented companies will need to jettison much of their bureaucracy since their competition for research discoveries will be smaller entrepreneurial corporations with greater flexibility to rapidly exploit the changing scientific environment. Consequently, entrepreneurial vigor among scientists will be a major determinant of the success of a given company. Obviously, developing a cadre of personnel with broad, "renaissance man" experiences and entrepreneurial vigor will be a major challenge for pharmaceutical companies.

D. Improvement of Quality

After all is said and done, the largest new opportunity is not terribly different from many old opportunities. We must improve quality. In this case, we must improve the quality of our research and the quality of our understanding and appreciation of what the resulting information enables. While this message seems simple, its implementation will not be easy. First and foremost, it runs counter to the trend toward a market-driven, short-term orientation. The extreme case of market drive is for a major pharmaceutical company to cease research operations and focus marketing efforts on an array of products acquired from smaller research-only companies. Some companies that approach this extreme case exist today. One component of this trend is growing as biotechnology companies continue to establish marketing relationships with major pharmaceutical companies.

V. THE THREE FACES OF THE FUTURE

The pharmaceutical industry may evolve into three segments, each with its own opportunities for profit centers. The first segment is pharmaceutical marketing and sales organizations. Some of the major pharmaceutical companies which had large M&S divisions in the late 1980s will ultimately become almost exclusively marketing and sales organizations. In this segment, the companies that retain any scientific divisions will concentrate principally on clinical drug development of new chemical entities acquired via licensure. Some drug discovery research may be undertaken in these organizations, but the majority of discovery expenditures will be directed towards discovery of compounds with predictable clinical utility based on prior experience in either the scientific or marketing community (i.e., so called "me-too" or "patented generic" compounds). This is analogous to what is occurring presently in the computer industry where many manufacturers attempt to mimic the capabilities of innovator companies. Further, both innovator and clone producer organizations are attempting to strike marketing arrangements with companies specializing in computer equipment, sales, and service.

The second segment consists of small science-driven research organizations that attempt to exploit their expertise in a particular technology or possibly in a particular therapeutic area to discover and develop innovative drugs, diagnostic products, and equipment useful for some medical sub-specialty. These organizations collectively will represent the major innovative force in the pharmaceutical industry. Again, using the computer industry analogy, these companies represent the organizations that satisfy the needs of selective market niches. Their marketing forces would certainly be minimal, if any. Marketing through a vendor company would be the essential means of moving their products into the marketplace. The number of companies in this segment will be large and their lifecycles may be volatile as technologies continue to change rapidly.

The third segment consists of the science-driven integrated pharmaceutical firms with broad scientific diversity in their drug discovery and development capabilities, as well as sophisticated M&S capabilities. These multinational organizations will clearly be the leaders and will market not only their own innovative products, but also products that they are able to license as a result of their scientific expertise. The number of companies in this segment will be quite small, probably less than ten. Their achievements of consistent long-term investment in R&D, high research equity, and maximum return on their research information bases will be the keys to earning them entry to this segment.

In all three segments of the industry, the greatest opportunities will be on the roads least traveled.

Index

215